# Register Now for Online Access to Your Book!

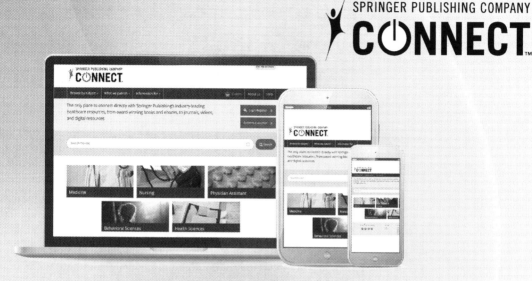

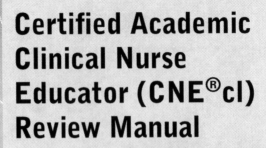

# Certified Academic
# Clinical Nurse
# Educator (CNE®cl)
# Review Manual

**Ruth A. Wittmann-Price, PhD, RN, CNS, CNE, CHSE, CNEcl, ANEF, FAAN**, is the founding dean of the School of Health Sciences at Francis Marion University, Florence, South Carolina. She received her BSN degree from Felician College in Lodi, New Jersey; her master's from Columbia University, New York, New York; and completed her PhD in nursing at Widener University, Chester, Pennsylvania, receiving the Dean's Award for Excellence. She developed a midrange nursing theory, "Emancipated Decision-Making in Women's Health Care," and has tested her theory in four studies. This theory recognizes that oppression continues to exist in the healthcare setting and is imposed by society for purposes of situational control affecting the decisions women make about healthcare for themselves and their families. The theory is referenced in multiple books and is being used in Asia, Africa, Brazil, Colombia, the United Kingdom, and Canada. The University of Limpopo, in South Africa, has applied the theory to the Community-Oriented Nursing Education Program for Women and Child Health (CONEWCH) project. This project institutes a community-oriented nursing education program to improve health of women and children. In her administrative role, Dr. Wittmann-Price has turned her attention to underserved students and has secured over $6 million in federal funding. Those funds are currently supporting disadvantaged nursing students to care for patients in the rural, underserved Pee Dee region of South Carolina. Dr. Wittmann-Price has authored over 16 books and numerous articles, and presents internationally and nationally.

**Linda Wilson, PhD, RN, CPAN, CAPA, BC, CNE, CHSE-A, CNEcl, FASPAN, ANEF, FAAN,** is an assistant dean for Continuing Education, Simulation and Events and a clinical professor in the Division of Nursing at Drexel University, College of Nursing and Health Professions in Philadelphia, Pennsylvania. Dr. Wilson completed her BSN at College Misericordia in Dallas, Pennsylvania, and completed her MSN in Critical Care and Trauma at Thomas Jefferson University in Philadelphia. She completed her PhD in nursing research at Rutgers University in Newark, New Jersey. Dr. Wilson also has a postgraduate certificate in epidemiology and biostatistical methods from Drexel University and a postgraduate certificate in pain management from the University of California San Francisco, School of Medicine. Dr. Wilson also completed the National Library of Medicine/Marine Biological Laboratory, Biomedical Informatics Fellowship and the Harvard University Institute for Medical Simulation's Comprehensive Workshop and Graduate Course in Medical Simulation. Dr. Wilson has several certifications: CPAN, CAPA, American Nurses Credentialing Center (ANCC) Board Certified in Nursing Professional Development (BC), CNE, CNEcl, CHSE-A. Dr. Wilson served as the president of the American Society of Perianesthesia Nurses (2002–2003) and as an ANCC Commission on Accreditation Appraiser site surveyor since 2000. Dr. Wilson was inducted as a fellow in the Academy of Nurse Educator Fellows (ANEF) and the American Academy of Nursing (FAAN) in 2014.

**Karen K. Gittings, DNP, RN, CNE, CNEcl, Alumnus CCRN,** is an associate professor of nursing, associate dean of the School of Health Sciences, chair of the nursing program, and director of the Master of Science in Nursing (MSN) Nurse Educator track at Francis Marion University, Florence, South Carolina. Dr. Gittings received her diploma in nursing from The Washington Hospital School of Nursing and her BSN from the University of Maryland, Baltimore County campus. She received her MSN with specialization in nursing education and her DNP from Duquesne University in Pittsburgh, Pennsylvania. She was a 2015 to 2016 Amy V. Cockcroft Fellow, achieved certification in online instruction in 2011, and became a Certified Nurse Educator (CNE) in 2013. Dr. Gittings has extensive experience in critical care nursing and has been a certified critical care RN (CCRN) since 1991. Her areas of teaching expertise are medical–surgical nursing, critical care, and cardiac nursing. She has taught both junior- and senior-level undergraduate, baccalaureate nursing students in the classroom and clinical settings, and graduate students in the nursing education track. Karen has published in *Medical–Surgical Nursing Test Success: An Unfolding Case Study Review*, and Med-Surg Q&A (an electronic application); she also contributed to two books, *Fast Facts for Developing a Nursing Academic Portfolio* and *Review Manual for the Certified Healthcare Simulation Educator™ (CHSE™) Exam*. Dr. Gittings has also presented nationally on the topics of intravenous education through simulation, developing an effective nurse educator academic portfolio for career growth and advancement, designing a full 8-hour simulation day, concept mapping, and teaching clinical decision-making. She is the immediate past president of Francis Marion University's Chi Lambda Chapter of Sigma Theta Tau International. She is past president of Francis Marion University's chapter of Phi Kappa Phi and the Pee Dee Area Chapter of the American Association of Critical-Care Nurses. She is a recipient of multiple Outstanding Faculty Teaching Awards at Francis Marion University and the South Carolina Palmetto Gold Award (2005).

# Certified Academic Clinical Nurse Educator (CNE®cl) Review Manual

**Ruth A. Wittmann-Price, PhD, RN, CNS, CNE, CHSE, CNEcl, ANEF, FAAN**

**Linda Wilson, PhD, RN, CPAN, CAPA, BC, CNE, CHSE-A, CNEcl, FASPAN, ANEF, FAAN**

**Karen K. Gittings, DNP, RN, CNE, CNEcl, Alumnus CCRN**

SPRINGER PUBLISHING COMPANY

Copyright © 2020 Springer Publishing Company, LLC

Springer Publishing Company, LLC
11 West 42nd Street
New York, NY 10036
www.springerpub.com
http://connect.springerpub.com

*Acquisitions Editor*: Margaret Zuccarini
*Compositor*: diacriTech

*ISBN*: 978-0-8261-9493-0
*ebook ISBN*: 978-0-8261-9494-7
*DOI:* 10.1891/9780826194947

19 20 21 22 23 / 5 4 3 2 1

The author and the publisher of this Work have made every effort to use sources believed to be reliable to provide information that is accurate and compatible with the standards generally accepted at the time of publication. Because medical science is continually advancing, our knowledge base continues to expand. Therefore, as new information becomes available, changes in procedures become necessary. We recommend that the reader always consult current research and specific institutional policies before performing any clinical procedure. The author and publisher shall not be liable for any special, consequential, or exemplary damages resulting, in whole or in part, from the readers' use of, or reliance on, the information contained in this book. The publisher has no responsibility for the persistence or accuracy of URLs for external or third-party Internet websites referred to in this publication and does not guarantee that any content on such websites is, or will remain, accurate or appropriate.

CNE®cl is a registered trademark of the National League for Nursing, which neither sponsors nor endorses this product.

**Library of Congress Cataloging-in-Publication Data**

Names: Wittmann-Price, Ruth A., author. | Wilson, Linda, 1962- author. | Gittings, Karen K., author.
Title: Certified academic clinical nurse educator (CNE®cl) review manual / Ruth A. Wittmann-Price, PhD, RN, CNS, CNE, CHSE, CNEcl, ANEF, FAAN Linda Wilson, PhD, RN, CPAN, CAPA, BC, CNE, CHSE-A, CNEcl, FASPAN, ANEF, FAAN Karen K. Gittings, DNP, RN, CNE, CNEcl, Alumnus CCRN.
Description: New York, NY : Springer Publishing Company, LLC, [2019] | Includes bibliographical references and index.
Identifiers: LCCN 2019015627| ISBN 9780826194930 | ISBN 9780826194947 (ebook)
Subjects: LCSH: Nursing schools–Faculty–Certification–Study guides. | Nursing–Practice–Examinations, questions, etc. | Nursing schools–Faculty–Vocational guidance. | Nursing–Study and teaching.
Classification: LCC RT90 .W57 2019 | DDC 610.73076–dc23 LC record available at
  https://lccn.loc.gov/2019015627

Contact us to receive discount rates on bulk purchases.
We can also customize our books to meet your needs.
For more information please contact: sales@springerpub.com

**Publisher's Note:** New and used products purchased from third-party sellers are not guaranteed for quality, authenticity, or access to any included digital components.

Printed in the United States of America.

*To my granddaughter, Alice Ruth Moyer.*
*—Ruth A. Wittmann-Price*

*To H. Lynn Kane, Helen "Momma" Kane, and Linda Webb, thank you for your amazing friendship and for being my family. To Lou Smith, Trisha Costa DePena, Steve Johnson, Evan Babcock, and Elizabeth Diaz, thank you for your friendship and support. To Nick Foles and the Philadelphia Eagles, thank you for inspiration.*
*—Linda Wilson*

*To my family with love.*
*—Karen K. Gittings*

# Contents

# Contributors

**Betty Abraham-Settles, DNP, RN-BC**   Assistant Professor, University of South Carolina School of Nursing, Aiken, South Carolina

**Tracy P. George, DNP, APRN-BC, CNE**   Assistant Professor of Nursing, Department of Nursing, Francis Marion University, Florence, South Carolina

**Karen K. Gittings, DNP, RN, CNE, CNEcl, Alumnus CCRN** Associate Dean, School of Health Sciences; Chair, Department of Nursing; and Associate Professor of Nursing, Francis Marion University, Florence, South Carolina

**Mary Ellen Smith Glasgow, PhD, RN, ACNS-BC, ANEF, FAAN** Dean and Professor, School of Nursing, Duquesne University, Pittsburgh, Pennsylvania

**Wendy H. Hatchell, MSN-Ed, RN**   Instructor of Nursing, Department of Nursing, Francis Marion University, Florence, South Carolina

**Marty Hucks, MN, APRN-BC, CNE**   Assistant Professor of Nursing, Department of Nursing, Francis Marion University, Florence, South Carolina

**M. Annie Muller, DNP, APRN-BC**   Associate Professor of Nursing, Department of Nursing, Francis Marion University, Florence, South Carolina

**Fabien Pampaloni, MSN, RN**   International Business Affairs Specialist for Pocket Nurse®, Monaca, Pennsylvania

**Dorie L. Weaver, DNP, FNP-BC, NE, CNE**   Assistant Professor of Nursing, Department of Nursing, Francis Marion University, Florence, South Carolina

**Demica N. Williams, MSN, RN, CNE** Clinical Nurse Educator for Intermediate Services, University Hospital, Augusta, Georgia

**Linda Wilson, PhD, RN, CPAN, CAPA, BC, CNE, CHSE-A, CNEcl, FASPAN, ANEF, FAAN**   Assistant Dean for Continuing Education, Simulation and Events, and Clinical Professor, Division of Nursing, College of Nursing and Health Professions, Drexel University, Philadelphia, Pennsylvania

**Ruth A. Wittmann-Price, PhD, RN, CNS, CNE, CHSE, CNEcl, ANEF, FAAN**   Dean, School of Health Sciences, and Professor of Nursing, Francis Marion University, Florence, South Carolina

# Foreword

Clinical nursing education is pivotal to the formation of a competent, ethical professional nurse who contributes to the health and well-being of patients across the nation and globe. Benner, Sutphen, Leonard, and Day (2010) indicated that knowledge acquisition, clinical integration, and ethical comportment are vital to the development of critical reasoning and professional development. Clinical nurse educators support students in gaining new competencies in a broad spectrum of skills, providing them challenges and opportunities to grow. However, the clinical component of nursing education is frequently not afforded the proper attribution and gravitas for its contributions to the development of the professional nurse.

I would like to acknowledge the National League for Nursing (NLN) for having the foresight to recognize the importance of the clinical nurse educator role by offering the Certified Academic Clinical Nurse Educator (CNE®cl) certification exam. The CNEcl exam has the potential to "raise the bar" with respect to clinical nursing education by drawing attention to clinical nurse educator knowledge and competencies.

Clinical nursing education today is incredibly complex, and every clinical nurse educator needs some familiarity with clinical education pedagogies and evaluation methods, clinical agency policy standards, and academic policies. Novice clinical nurse educators face a particularly steep learning curve and new challenges as they enter the academy, and even more so if their graduate education did not have specific coursework on the teaching role. Clinical pedagogy, simulation, clinical evaluation, academic culture, progression policies, and legal considerations with respect to student conduct and academic and clinical appeals are among the areas that the clinical nurse educator needs to learn and eventually master.

Learning occurs if the role model is relevant, credible, and knowledgeable. In the context of the clinical environment, students benefit from clinical nurse educators who have the expert knowledge, interpersonal skills, credibility, and authority, leading to knowledge acquisition and empowerment.

It is my hope that clinical nurse educators take pride in this critical role in nursing education, develop their craft to its fullest potential, and receive the proper acknowledgment for their knowledge and skills through NLN certification.

*Mary Ellen Smith Glasgow, PhD, RN, ACNS-BC, ANEF, FAAN*
Dean and Professor
Duquesne University

## ▦ REFERENCE

Benner, P., Sutphen, M., Leonard, V., & Day, L. (2010). *Educating nurses: A call for radical transformation*. San Francisco, CA: Jossey-Bass/Carnegie Foundation for the Advancement of Teaching.

# Preface

Nurse educators are an amazing group of scholars who possess two areas of expertise: nursing education and a clinical specialty. Clinical nurse educators are the "boots on the ground" in the development of nursing professionals. The National League for Nursing's (NLN's) Certified Academic Clinical Nurse Educator examination (CNE®cl; NLN, 2018) is a mark of excellence for nurse educators who teach in the clinical learning environment (CLE; Barbe & Kimble, 2018).

This book was developed by expert nurse educators in academia and clinical practice to assist others in obtaining wanted certification (Lundeen, 2018). Chapter 1, CNE®cl Exam Specifics, helps readers grasp the parameters of the examination. Chapter 2, Test-Taking Strategies, reviews test-taking strategies because even though nurse educators teach, when anyone is placed back into the student role, a review assists him or her to apply concepts to themselves. Chapter 3 (Functioning Within the Education and Healthcare Environments: Function in the Clinical Educator Role), Chapter 4 (Functioning Within the Education and Healthcare Environments: Operationalize the Curriculum), and Chapter 5 (Functioning Within the Education and Healthcare Environments: Abide by Legal Requirements, Ethical Guidelines, Agency Policies, and Guiding Framework) address aspects of functioning within the education and healthcare environments. Chapter 3 begins to address the scope of the content outline within the test plan by reviewing the clinical nurse educator role. Chapter 4 operationalizes the curriculum and describes the process of transference of knowledge from classroom to patient care. Chapter 5 reviews legal and ethical issues faced by clinical nurse educators in the increasingly complex healthcare system. Chapter 6, Facilitate Learning in the Healthcare Environment, describes the learning process experienced within the clinical environment, and Chapter 7, Demonstrate Effective Interpersonal Communication and Collaborative Interprofessional Relationships, addresses interprofessional relationships. Interprofessional relationship development is key to maintaining patient safety for all healthcare students. The focus of Chapter 8, Apply Clinical Expertise in the Healthcare Environment, is clinical expertise and how the clinical nurse educator can incorporate expertise to enhance and expand student learning opportunities. Chapter 9, Facilitate Learner Development and Socialization, describes student socialization, an important consideration for all nurse educators when educating healthcare professionals. Chapter 10, Implement Effective Clinical Assessment and Evaluation Strategies, reviews the parameters of student assessment and evaluation within the CLE.

It is important to note that although this review provides practice questions and case studies at the end of each chapter, Chapter 11 offers an entire practice test and Chapter 12 provides answers and rationales to these practice questions, which are designed to prepare you for the CNEcl examination. Our hope is that this book will support you during your journey toward certification to help you achieve recognition of the critically important work you do in shaping the next generation of nursing professionals. We wish you the very best of luck.

*Ruth A. Wittmann-Price*
*Linda Wilson*
*Karen K. Gittings*

## ▓ REFERENCES

Barbe, T., & Kimble, L. P. (2018). What is the value of nurse education certification? A comparison study of certified and noncertified nurse educators. *Nursing Education Perspective, 39*(2), 66–71. doi: 10.1097/01.NEP.0000000000000261

Lundeen, J. D. (2018). Analysis of first-time unsuccessful attempts on the Certified Nurse Educator examination. *Nursing Education Perspective, 39*(2), 72–78. doi:10.1097/01.NEP.0000000000000276

National League for Nursing. (2018). *Certified Academic Clinical Nurse Educator (CNE®cl) 2018 candidate handbook.* Retrieved from http://www.nln.org/docs/default-source/testing-services/CNEcl-handbook-jan-2018.docx?sf

# 1

# CNE®CL Exam Specifics

*FABIEN PAMPALONI*

> *Education is not preparation for life; education is life itself.*
> —John Dewey

## ■ LEARNING OUTCOMES

At the end of this chapter, the learner will be able to

- Discuss the importance of preparing and taking the Certified Academic Clinical Nurse Educator (CNE®cl) certification examination.
- Demonstrate understanding of the examination's structure.
- Integrate core competencies into clinical practice to evaluate self-effectiveness.

## ■ INTRODUCTION

The Certified Academic Clinical Nurse Educator (CNEcl) certification examination was created in order to verify the expertise of clinical nurse educators in the roles assigned to them by nursing programs (e.g., adjunct faculty, clinical instructor, or preceptor). With the responsibility of facilitating student learning through clinical experiences, educators obtaining the CNEcl will demonstrate the ability to effectively evaluate students' performances in reaching expected learning outcomes (National League for Nursing [NLN], 2018). The CNEcl examination comes at a good time, as the ever-growing nurse educator shortage is affecting the nation's workforce with increasing force. According to a 2016 to 2017 survey from the American Association of Colleges of Nursing (AACN), U.S. baccalaureate and graduate nursing schools have turned away 64,067 qualified applicants from programs due to insufficient faculty members, clinical placements, clinical faculty, and preceptors (AACN, 2017). The AACN (2017) study urges nursing programs to not only produce new nursing educators, but also to entice veteran clinical nurses to become educators in order to guarantee quality and effective knowledge transfer based on extensive and reliable experience.

## WHY BECOME A CNECL-CERTIFIED EDUCATOR?

*Certification* is defined by the American Board of Nursing Specialties (ABNS) as the formal recognition of specialized skills, knowledge, and experience demonstrated by the achievement of standards identified by a nursing specialty to promote optimal health outcomes (ABNS, 2016, p.1). Certification is a method that clinical nurse educators can use to validate their knowledge, skills, and experience beyond their initial licensure (Haskins, Hnatiuk, & Yoder, 2011; Hines, 2012; Miller, 2012). The 2018 National League for Nursing's CNEcl handbook emphasizes many certification benefits. From becoming an educational leader and role model to recognizing the nursing education profession as a specialty area of practice, the CNEcl certification demonstrates to students, faculty, and the community that the highest standards of excellence are being met (NLN, 2018). These benefits are aligned with goals that guarantee an all-inclusive and excellent knowledge transfer between the certified nurse educator and students. These goals are as follows:

- Distinguish academic clinical nursing education as a specialty area of practice.
- Recognize the academic clinical nurse educator's specialized knowledge, skills and abilities, and excellence in clinical teaching.
- Strengthen the use of selected core competencies of academic clinical nurse educator practice.
- Contribute to academic clinical nurse educators' professional development (NLN, 2018).

## WHAT IS THE VALUE OF CERTIFICATION?

The reasons why one chooses to become certified vary tremendously. These reasons may be driven by intrinsic or extrinsic factors. It may be a requirement for employment or one may simply choose to become certified for her or his own self-fulfillment. Specialty certification validates one's knowledge and expertise, builds confidence and credibility, and demonstrates dedication to the nursing profession (extrinsic and intrinsic factors are expanded in Chapter 3, Functioning Within the Education and Healthcare Environments: Function in the Clinical Educator Role). Benefits of certification may include personal growth, professional development, career advancement, tangible financial incentives, and perceived empowerment. Individuals are motivated toward a goal by their values. If you value certification as an essential component of your career, then you most likely will decide to work on achieving this goal (Schroeter, 2015).

## ▪ CORE COMPETENCIES FOR NURSE EDUCATORS

In order to ensure effective knowledge transfer, the NLN has developed core competencies that are used as evaluation guides for the clinical nurse educators' effectiveness. Table 1.1 describes how core competencies are applied by faculty in the clinical environment.

| Table 1.1 Clinical Applications in Meeting the NLN Core Competencies | |
|---|---|
| **Competency** | **Clinical Applications** |
| Facilitate learning | • Serve as a positive role model of professional nursing by exhibiting characteristics such as being empathetic, supportive, nonjudgmental, calm, and approachable.<br>• Demonstrate passion for teaching, learning, and the field of nursing to inspire and motivate learners.<br>• Clinical experiences should give the learners opportunities to apply content they learned in the classroom and perform skills practiced in the laboratory.<br>• Initial experiences should involve basic care (bathing, ambulating) and then progress to more complex skills (suctioning, wound care, intravenous therapy).<br>• Ask the learners questions about the care they are giving and expected results of patient treatments.<br>• Implement varied clinical teaching models. |
| Facilitate learner development and socialization | • Provide a learning environment that fosters cognitive, psychomotor, and affective learning.<br>• Promote professional integrity, accountability, and emphasize maintaining respect and dignity for all.<br>• Help students engage in a self-reflection process that helps them identify their goals and limitations, and to establish ways to improve their practice. |

*(continued)*

| Table 1.1 Clinical Applications in Meeting the NLN Core Competencies *(continued)* | |
| --- | --- |
| **Competency** | **Clinical Applications** |
| | • Foster professional growth of learners through coaching, simulation experiences, and debriefing. |
| | • Maintain professional boundaries. |
| | • Engage learners in applying best practices. |
| | • Plan appropriate clinical learning activities to promote clinical decision-making and teamwork. |
| | • Apply ethical and legal principles to ensure a safe learning environment. |
| | • Adhere to program and clinical agency policies, procedures, and standards of practice. |
| | • Create an environment that focuses on preparing learners for their future roles. |
| | • Familiarize learners with the various cultural beliefs that could impact the way they deliver nursing care. |
| | • Identify learners who are not adjusting well to their role as a future nurse and advise and counsel them as necessary. |
| Use assessment and evaluation strategies | • Use a variety of strategies to assess and evaluate learners' abilities to meet course outcomes. These data also should be used to enhance the teaching/learning process. |
| | • Provide timely, constructive, objective, and fair written feedback to learners. |
| | • Be precise and specific when providing constructive criticism. Criticism should identify specific areas of strengths and weaknesses. |
| | • Maintain timely communication with course faculty regarding learner performance and progression. |
| | • Assess congruency and quality of clinical agency to the course goals and learner needs. |
| Participate in curriculum design and evaluation of program outcomes | • Clinical nurse educators can contribute to curriculum development and program evaluation based on their current practice. Practicing in a clinical setting keeps one up to date on current healthcare delivery trends as well as with the roles and responsibilities of nurses working within a consistently changing environment. |
| | • Clinical nurse educator experience can help to identify learner competencies that address current societal and healthcare trends. |

*(continued)*

**Table 1.1 Clinical Applications in Meeting the NLN Core Competencies** (*continued*)

| Competency | Clinical Applications |
|---|---|
| Function as a change agent and leader | • Value interprofessional communication and collaboration along with emphasizing the importance of a shared learning environment.<br>• Clinical nurse educators participate in interprofessional efforts to address healthcare and educational needs.<br>• Active involvement on an advisory board promotes collegial efforts between the nursing program and the partnering healthcare agencies to support educational goals.<br>• Teach and encourage the process of quality improvement.<br>• Discuss and display effective conflict management.<br>• Demonstrate effective leadership qualities. |
| Pursue continuous quality improvement in the nurse educator role | • To advance, learners need to be provided with opportunities for professional development.<br>• Use a patient-centered approach to clinical instruction.<br>• Use technology (educational resources, electronic health records) to support the teaching–learning process. |
| Engage in scholarship | • Demonstrate that nursing standards are grounded in evidence-based practice.<br>• Assign a project that explores the research literature regarding a specific skill or treatment intervention to foster a spirit of inquiry and introduce learners to the concept of evidence-based practice.<br>• Maintain current professional competence relevant to the specialty area and CLE.<br>• Clinical nurse educators must maintain a commitment to lifelong learning (formal education, continuing-education programs, and/or certification). |
| Function within the educational environment | • Emphasize the significance of belonging to a nursing organization, such as the National Student Nurses' Association. This can help students learn the importance of developing networks with others in the nursing profession. |
|  | • Discuss the benefits of continued membership within professional organizations, such as helping to assume leadership roles and being healthcare advocates within the political arena. |

CLE, clinical learning environment; NLN, National League for Nursing.
*Source:* Fressola, M. C., & Patterson, G. E. (2017). *Transition from clinician to educator: A practical approach.* Burlington, MA: Jones & Bartlett Learning.

## ▦ TEST PREREQUISITES

Although many educators are eager to obtain such recognized certification, some eligibility requirements have to be met in order to qualify for testing. The requirements are based on past educational and professional experience and are described in Table 1.2.

| Table 1.2 Requirements for Testing | |
| --- | --- |
| **Option A: Must meet criteria 1, 2, and 3** | **Option B: Must meet criteria 1, 2, 3, and 4** |
| 1. Licensure: Documentation of valid licensure/certificate or other documentation of unencumbered practice as a nurse in one's country of residence | 1. Licensure: Documentation of valid licensure/certificate or other documentation of unencumbered practice in one's country of residence |
| 2. Education: A graduate degree with a focus in nursing education | 2. Education: A baccalaureate degree in nursing (or higher) |
| 3. Professional Practice: Three years working in any area of nursing | 3. Professional Practice: Three years experience in any area of nursing |
| | 4. Academic Practice: Two years of teaching experience in an academic setting within the last 5 years (may include simulation) |

*Source:* National League for Nursing. (2018). *Certified Academic Clinical Nurse Educator (CNE®cl) 2018 candidate handbook.* Retrieved from http://www.nln.org/docs/default-source/default-document-library/cnecl-handbook-jan-2018.pdf?sfvrsn=4

## ▦ TEST STRUCTURE

The CNEcl examination is composed of 150 multiple-choice items with a total of 130 questions counting toward the actual test score. The remaining 20 questions or items are currently being tested for validity and reliability and will not count toward the final test results. These latter items are unknown to the test-taker and will be used for further test improvements if results are satisfactory (NLN, 2018). Educators who decided to take the CNEcl examination are tested in six major content areas: function within the education and healthcare environments (19%), facilitate learning in the healthcare environment (19%), demonstrate effective interpersonal communication and collaborative interprofessional relationships (15%), application of clinical expertise in the healthcare environment (15%), facilitate learner development and socialization (15%), and implement effective clinical assessment and evaluation strategies (17%). These content areas are reflected within the test and the test-taker is challenged to know the content areas in three cognitive levels:

• Recall

• Application

• Analysis (NLN, 2018; these domains are expanded in Chapter 2, Test-Taking Strategies).

The pilot examination for the CNEcl was completed late in 2018. Sixty nurse educators took the examination during the NLN Summit in Chicago, whereas others took the examination online. All first-time test-takers were notified of their scores by mid-October 2018. The pass rate was 86% and the cut score was determined. Of the 130 functional questions, an educator needs 92 correct answers to pass. Results are now provided immediately after the test is completed at the testing center.

The certification is granted for a duration of 5 years and renewal is offered to clinical nurse educators who have maintained practice and professional requirements. Clinical nurse educators can submit evidence that practice and professional requirements have been maintained or retake the CNEcl examination. Audits are possible during the certification renewal process in order to guarantee the ongoing integrity of the evidence submitted for recertification (NLN, 2018).

A detailed breakdown of all the content areas is available at www.nln.org/docs/default-source/default-document-library/cnecl-handbook-jan-2018.pdf?sfvrsn=4.

## ▪ SUMMARY

Clinical nurse educators take an immense pride in their professional and educational accomplishments. Certifications, such as the CNEcl, reflect achievements and a strong dedication to the nursing profession. As indicated in the troublesome study mentioned at the beginning of this chapter regarding the nursing faculty shortage, turning away new nursing students because of a lack of faculty cannot become a new norm in the industry. Becoming a CNEcl-certified clinical nurse educator will not only help solve the nursing faculty challenge but also ensure that quality nurses are graduating who can efficiently provide the best patient care.

## ▪ REFERENCES

American Academy of Colleges of Nursing. (2017). *Nursing faculty shortage fact sheet*. Retrieved from https://www.aacnnursing.org/Portals/42/News/Factsheets/Faculty-Shortage-Factsheet-2017.pdf

American Board of Nursing Specialties. (2016). *About us: Our history*. Retrieved from http://www.nursingcertification.org/about

Fressola, M. C., & Patterson, G. E. (2017). *Transition from clinician to educator: A practical approach*. Burlington, MA: Jones & Bartlett Learning.

Haskins, M., Hnatiuk, C., & Yoder, L. (2011). Medical–surgical nurses' perceived value of certification study. *Medical–Surgical Nurses, 20*(2), 71–77.

Hines, M. E. (2012). The value of specialty nursing certification for holistic nurses. *American Holistic Nurses, 32*(1), 12–19.

Miller, K. (2012). From the certified board nurse life care planning, licensure, specialty designation, certification, & accreditation. *Journal of Nurse Life Care Planning, 12*(4), 735–737.

National League for Nursing. (2018). *Certified Academic Clinical Nurse Educator (CNE®cl) 2018 candidate handbook*. Retrieved from http://www.nln.org/docs/default-source/default-document-library/cnecl-handbook-jan-2018.pdf?sfvrsn=4

Schroeter, K. (2015). The value of certification. *Journal of Trauma Nursing, 22*(2), 53–54. doi:10.1097/JTN.0000000000000120

# 2

# Test-Taking Strategies

DORIE L. WEAVER

*Always walk through life as if you have something new to learn
and you will.*
—Vernon Howard

## ■ LEARNING OUTCOMES

At the end of this chapter, the learner will be able to

1. Discover the process to best prepare for the certification examination.
2. Organize and design a realistic study plan to help prepare for the Certified Academic Clinical Nurse Educator (CNE®cl) examination.
3. Execute strategies to reduce test anxiety.
4. Demonstrate adequate time-management skills to enhance studying.
5. Integrate individual learning styles to promote learning.

## ■ INTRODUCTION

According to the U.S. Bureau of Labor Statistics (2018), positions for RNs are expected to grow by 15% between 2016 and 2026. This growth is predicted to occur for various reasons, including an increased emphasis on health promotion; growing rates of chronic diseases among all age groups; and the rise in demand for healthcare within the baby boom population, the members of which are living longer and more active lives. In addition, the Institute of Medicine (IOM) supports the fact that a more highly educated nursing workforce is critical for patients to receive safe and effective care (IOM, 2010). The IOM recommendation calls for at least 80% of the RN workforce to be prepared at the baccalaureate level by 2020.

With this increase in need for baccalaureate-prepared RNs, there comes an increased need for nurse educators. The U.S. Bureau of Labor Statistics (2018) reports that the average annual salary of a nurse educator is $77,360, and employment in the field is projected to grow 24% between 2016 and 2026. Educational institutions are struggling to fill faculty positions with qualified educators to meet this demand. This shortage can be seen among academic and clinical nurse educators alike, resulting in qualified students getting turned away from nursing programs.

## ▓ THE ROLE OF THE CLINICAL NURSE EDUCATOR

Nurse educators play an invaluable role in preparing students to enter the healthcare field. They have a colossal responsibility to ensure learners are well equipped to perform safely within a wide array of clinical settings. Clinical faculty play an equally vital role in a learner's education. Their role is to teach the learner how to transfer the knowledge learned in the classroom and to apply it while caring for patients.

| 2.1 Clinical Nurse Educator Teaching Tip |
| --- |
| The passion you demonstrate on the clinical unit is easily perceived by students and can influence their learning. |

The role of a nurse is dynamic; therefore, clinical nurse educators must be flexible by acknowledging changes to the system and sharing this new information with their learners. They must be willing to move past former beliefs and practices in favor of new requirements that learners will deal with in the workforce. Clinical nurse educators need not only to be well versed in nursing, but also in education. This includes knowledge of overarching concepts behind the learning process, such as varied theories, learning styles, pedagogical methodologies, and evaluative strategies (Fressola & Patterson, 2017).

| 2.1 Evidence-Based Clinical Teaching Practice |
| --- |
| Students' satisfaction with clinical learning improved when faculty made clear assignments, provided specific instructions, maintained organization, and provided individualized attention (Lovecchio, DiMattio, & Hudacek, 2015). |

| 2.2 Clinical Nurse Educator Teaching Tip |
|---|
| Just as no two patients are alike, the same goes for students. What works for one student may not work for another. A nurse educator must be able to convey knowledge using a variety of methods in order to meet the needs of her or his students. |

## ◼ LEARNING STYLES

Recognizing your personal learning preferences can maximize your clinical teaching strengths. This is referred to as your *learning style,* or the way you take in and processinformation. Perhaps you get more out of studying with others than you do by studying alone (Blevins, 2014). The process of identifying your learning and study preferences can be very powerful. It can help you develop strategies to help you study more effectively. There are a number of instruments available to help you understand your learning style to guide your study methods. Knowing how you learn will help you set and achieve specific goals. The one instrument discussed in this chapter is the VARK questionnaire. The acronym *VARK* is based on four sensory modalities: visual, aural/auditory, read/write, and kinesthetic (VARK®, n.d.). This questionnaire can be accessed online at www.vark-learn.com/the-vark-questionnaire.

After you take the VARK questionnaire, you will receive a score that tabulates how many questions you answered that correspond to each sensory modality. You may have two or more modalities with similar scores, which is referred to as *multimodal*. The visual (V) learner prefers to use images such as charts, pictures, diagrams, timelines, symbols, and maps. These learners prefer symbols that exhibit patterns or demonstrate correlation. Such symbols help make meaningful connections to words (Shushan, 2017). A good way to learn a topic may be by creating a concept map or using computer graphics. During study sessions, it would be handy to draw visual representations of the information along with using symbols to make associations. Creating concept maps would be a great assignment for visual learners. Concept maps are a teaching–learning strategy in which a diagram is used to connect concepts. Concept maps have been found effective in developing critical thinking skills (Chan, 2017).

The aural/auditory (A) learner focuses on listening to what is heard or spoken. The auditory learner may learn best by listening to recorded lectures, tutorials, group discussions, web chats, podcasts, and speaking aloud the content that is being studied. Reading important details aloud can be beneficial in sorting concepts and to gain understanding. In addition, teaching concepts to others within a study group can be helpful. Auditory learners can also ask a study group member to quiz them on the material (Fleming, 2001).

The read/write (R) learner prefers to learn using written words whether by the act of writing or act of reading. These students learn by writing notes that highlight important points. In addition, they like to write material in their own words to enhance their understanding (Shushan, 2017). Students who prefer this method like PowerPoint, the Internet, lists, dictionaries, thesauri, quotations, and anything with words (Fleming, 2001).

The kinesthetic (K) learner has a preference for hands-on, real-world learning that has a physical component. This can include simulation or involve real practice experiences. These individuals learn best when they are doing something physical to learn a concept or by watching a live demonstration as they experience learning in a concrete way. Kinesthetic learners gain a better understanding of material when they use their bodies and engage one or more of their senses (Fleming, 2001). Study methods that may be beneficial for this type of learner would be using virtual simulations, role playing, or gaming.

There are numerous ways to study. To increase your understanding of material and to ensure your success on the certification exam, determine what study techniques might complement your VARK preference(s). You may study most effectively by using flash cards, rewriting your notes, acting out scenarios, drawing visuals, or discussing material with study group members. Play to your strengths: Choose the study techniques that most align with your learning preference (Shushan, 2017).

## ▨ TYPES OF QUESTIONS DEVELOPED FROM THE COGNITIVE LEVELS OF LEARNING

Bloom's taxonomy of learning is used to determine whether the candidate has mastered definitive skills or competencies (Wilson & Wittmann-Price, 2015). Within the cognitive domain, objectives are divided into six levels, ranging from simple to complex. The certification examination reflects three of those six levels. The first level of questioning consists of recall. This is the ability to recall or recognize specific concepts. These types of questions are the least emphasized on the certification examination due to their uncomplicated nature (National League for Nursing [NLN], 2018).

The two remaining cognitive levels that will be highly emphasized on the CNEcl examination include application and analysis questions. Application questions expect the candidate to possess the ability to comprehend, relate, or apply ideas, concepts, principles, or theories to new or changing situations (NLN, 2018). These questions expect the candidate to provide an intervention to a problem. Analysis questions expect one to analyze, synthesize, and evaluate information. Analyzing information provides an opportunity to break down the relationship between the parts and decide how the whole functions. Ask yourself why a solution worked or didn't work. Your conclusion should always be supported by facts or results. Keep this in mind while you study for the certification exam. Although not used as frequently in testing situations, synthesis questions provide the opportunity to combine all elements into a unified whole to develop a tool or design a plan to create solutions to problems. In addition, evaluation will also be tested to provide the candidate with the opportunity to make value judgments based on the effectiveness of a clinical/simulation experience, case scenario progression, or patient outcomes using the interventions that were implemented (NLN, 2018).

The psychomotor domain of Bloom's taxonomy involves the ability of the student to properly execute gross and fine motor skills. When coupled with the cognitive domain, students understand the reason why the skill or action is being taken. By combining the two, the student is doing more than simply memorizing procedural steps. Finally, the affective domain includes learners' feelings, attitudes, and values. This includes the motivation to learn and the student's perception of the overall learning environment. Encouraging students to engage in reflection is a beneficial evaluation method within this domain because it is one that is not easily quantified. This method can assist students to clarify values, identify biases, and work through ethical dilemmas (McDonald, 2018).

## ▪ SETTING UP A STUDY PLAN

To increase one's success on the certification examination, advanced planning is extremely crucial. The best way to maximize your performance on this examination is to be certain to do three things: prepare, stay organized, and practice. One of the major pitfalls students face is failing to set aside adequate time to prepare. Prior to securing an examination date, ensure that there is sufficient time to study all concepts. A myth related to standardized examinations is that it is possible to unwrap the "tricks" of the exam; thereby enabling test-takers to perform well whether or not they know the information the questions are asking about. This is inaccurate because these exams are testing your knowledge base related to specific topics. There is no magic tactic you can use to succeed with this certification. One must come prepared with the essential knowledge.

Part of effective examination preparation involves "demystifying" the test design. It is crucial that candidates log into the NLN website to print the *Certified Academic Clinical Nurse Educator (CNE®cl) Candidate Handbook* (2018) (www.nln.org/docs/default-source/default-document-library/CNEcl-handbook-jan-2018.pdf?sfvrsn=4). The more familiar one is with the overall certification examination, the higher one's confidence level. Keeping the knowledge related to test design and blueprint in mind, it is now time to think about planning an effective study strategy. It is important tocreate a realistic, organized, and purposeful study plan to keep on track.

Create a weekly calendar and first insert time frames for all of your demands, including work hours, family, personal and professional commitments. After this has been completed, fill in the empty time slots available for studying. Make these times your study periods, and make them very visible by using color to highlight them. Remember that each week will have its own challenges so every week will differ. Fine-tune your schedule to accommodate your needs that week. You may need to subtract time in one place but add it in another. You may find you have more study time on weekends. In addition, do not forget to treat yourself and to take breaks.

You must be able to effectively manage and prioritize your time. Designate more time for areas that you have identified as weaknesses. Be certain you have allocated enough time to cover all examination content areas according to the blueprint. Because you cannot fully control time, it may be necessary to reschedule study time when a day has been particularly difficult. Trying to study when exhausted or distracted by other influences is basically counterproductive. In addition, it is vital to eliminate internal sources of distraction, such as fatigue, pain, hunger, or thirst. Minimizing distractions will maximize your concentration.

Set aside longer periods of time to study concepts that are more complex and those that carry the highest percentage of questions on the examination. Remaining organized includes creating a transparent, targeted study plan for the weeks leading up to the exam. Realize that NONE of this will work unless you believe in it, are realistic about your schedule, and stick with it! Think about when you study best (the more awake and alert you are, the better your concentration and focus will be). You may be a morning or evening person. In addition, think about where you study best (library, coffee shop, bedroom, or kitchen). Do you need complete silence or do you like a certain amount of noise?

What about exercise, which is SO VERY important? Slot in time for that. Exercise is a great way to boost your energy level as well as clear your mind. Also, if you plan for it in your schedule, you will not feel guilty about having fun. Remember that lack of sleep can contribute to memory loss and a lack of concentration. It is essential to obtain adequate sleep throughout your study schedule and definitely the evening prior to your scheduled examination. If you begin to feel anxious or overwhelmed, perform a chosen relaxation technique.

It is essential that you eat healthy foods during this process, so remember to schedule meal times. Be smart about your food choices: Think energy and brain power. You do not want to crash and burn! Avoid excessive amounts of caffeine, which can add to anxious feelings. Eat a light but nourishing meal that contains complex carbohydrates, fruits, vegetables, and high-quality protein to feed the mind and body. Consuming refined sugars and excessive fat intake can sap energy and derail study quality. Keep your body hydrated by drinking at least eight glasses of water each day. Also, remember that your emotional health is just as important as your physical health to promote learning and reduce anxiety. Make sure you set aside time for some social interaction with friends and family.

If you play an instrument or are on a sports team, you know that skill and comfort level improve the more you practice. The same benefits apply to test-taking. Practice answering questions on a routine basis. This helps learners to self-identify strengths and areas for improvement. Review the rationales that accompany practice questions regardless of whether you answered them correctly. These rationales may provide additional information you can apply to other questions. For those questions that you got wrong, take the time to research more about that content. Review the list of references on examination preparation and read multiple articles related to any category or concept for which you need more information (Wittmann-Price et al., 2017).

Practice exams should contain the same type of questions the certification exam does, they should be taken in situations that mimic the surroundings, and follow the time frame of the exam. This practice will help you be become more accustomed to sitting and maintaining focus for a sustained period of time. It will also help you learn how to pace yourself so that you do not have to rush at the end of the examination to beat the clock. Periodically check the time to determine whether you are progressing at an acceptable rate, and decide on a set number of questions that should be answered within a certain time period.

Self-Assessment Examination (SAE) is available to help prepare candidates for success in obtaining the CNEcl credential. This is an Internet-based, 65-item, multiple-choice practice exam offered by the NLN. The SAE can be used both as a learning tool and an assessment instrument. The SAE provides practice questions, which will help to increase comfort in computer-based tests, provides rationales for correct and incorrect answers, and a score report is made available to identify strengths and areas that need further improvement. The SAE is not intended to replace studying, but serves as an additional resource (NLN, 2018).

When studying, some people work best alone, whereas others benefit from collaborating with a study group. Study groups can be beneficial in sharing information and resources. To prevent the study group from getting off task, specific guidelines need to be formulated. It is vital that everyone is similarly committed. The meetings need a start and stop time as well as a set topic to discuss and predetermined learning objectives or outcomes for each session. Study groups work best when a group member serves as the leader for that session and leads the discussion on the particular topic of the day. This individual is also responsible for keeping the discussion on track and facilitating the efficient use of time and resources. Each person should be assigned a role and do some preparation in advance of the study session. Breaks can be taken but should be planned.

Additional study tips include the following:

- Organize information into groups.
- Use the concept of deep learning by critically examining new facts and making links between ideas.
- Relate new knowledge with existing knowledge.
- Use visual aids that will allow you to review information at a glance.
- Develop mnemonics as memory aids for specific material (Wittmann-Price et al., 2017).

Approaching examination day with an empowered and positive mind-set can help alleviate fears and keep the candidate confident. Visit the website of the certifying body to learn all that you can about test center rules, what you are and are not allowed to bring to the testing sites, and information about breaks and snacks. Leave yourself plenty of time to arrive at the test center to get settled. Perform a trial run so you can estimate how much time it will take you to travel there. Although the center attempts to make the environment as conducive for test-taking as possible, the reality is that not all aspects can be controlled. For example, someone could have a cough or the temperature may not be set to your preference. Dress in comfortable clothes and in layers so you are prepared for either warm or cool rooms.

## ▦ BASIC TESTING TIPS

- Make sure you read and understand the instructions.
- Read each question carefully and understand exactly what it is asking.
- Read all answer choices before making a selection. Avoid rapid guessing.
- Pace yourself and do not spend too much time on any one particular question.
- Only change answers when you are certain you chose the incorrect option. Be aware that the first choice is frequently the correct one.
- Be certain you provided an answer for every question. The examination will let you know how many questions were answered. If you have time and did not answer every question, go back and do so. Remember, there is no penalty for guessing and it increases your chances of being successful.
- Improve your odds of answering the question correctly by eliminating any incorrect choices.
- Identify key words or phrases within the question that may help guide you to the correct answer.

- Relate the content in the question to your experience as an educator and in practice. Previous experiences can be beneficial in answering questions.

- Remain calm if you are given a few consecutive questions that were very difficult, tell yourself these are experimental questions and will not count against you. You are not expected to answer every question correctly so enter the examination mentally prepared to encounter questions for which you do not know the answer.

## ■ COMBATING TEST ANXIETY

A certain level of anxiety can be beneficial. It can serve as a motivator and help the test-taker maintain focus during the examination. However, when anxiety becomes excessive, it can contribute to both physical and emotional symptoms, such as a rapid heartbeat, nausea, inability to concentrate due to racing thoughts, or feelings of fear or anger. Text anxiety can interfere with one's ability to think critically and disrupt performance during an exam situation.

Although it is completely normal to feel a bit nervous before an exam, test anxiety can be debilitating. Some causes of test anxiety may include a fear of failure, lack of adequate preparation time, negative experiences taking tests in the past, or not having recent test-taking experience. Following are a number of coping strategies that can be employed to ease test anxiety (Sawchuk, 2017):

- Adequate Preparation. Make sure you familiarize yourself with the content and types of questions on the exam along with the time allotted to complete the exam. Cramming is rarely a good study strategy and will only increase anxiety. It does not give your brain enough time to fully retain the material. It is important to study over the course of a few days or weeks to make sure you fully comprehend the material. Practice questions will help boost your confidence level.

- Watch Self-Talk. Take time to examine and challenge any negative thoughts. Write down every negative thought that has crossed your mind related to test-taking. Replace each of these with positive thoughts that argue against the negative one. Whenever negative thoughts intrude your mind, remind yourself of the positive ones. Another method used to improve positive thoughts is to repeat phrases such as "I can definitely do this." Visualize yourself doing well on the exam. This can help you make it happen in real life.

- Use Relaxation Techniques. To assist in helping clear your mind and stay calm before and during the examination, perform relaxation techniques such as deep breathing, progressive muscle relaxation, and guided imagery. These should be used days or weeks prior to the exam. The simple act of concentrating on these relaxation techniques as they are being performed can reduce or alleviate those uncomfortable anxiety-related feelings.

- Fuel Up. Your brain needs fuel to function. Eat a nutritious meal and drink plenty of water before the examination. Look for foods that offer a steady stream of nutrients. Avoid sugary drinks and snacks, which can cause your blood sugar to peak and then drop. Also avoid caffeinated beverages, such as coffee or energy drinks, which can increase anxiety.

- Regular Exercise. Aerobic exercise can release tension and keep stress to a minimum.

- Get Plenty of Sleep. Adequate sleep/rest is directly related to academic performance. A good night's sleep is necessary for optimal work performance.

- Arrive Early. Feeling rushed will only elevate your anxiety level. Get everything you need together the evening before the examination. Arrive at least 15 minutes early.

- Leisure Time. Engage in activities that bring you happiness and relaxation the evening prior to the examination, such as going out to dinner with family or friends or watching a movie or play. Last-minute studying will increase anxiety as most people begin to feel they have not studied enough and begin to doubt their readiness.

---

**2.2 Evidence-Based Clinical Teaching Practice**

A higher self-concept was found to be directly related to greater academic achievement. Test anxiety and intrinsic motivation were found to be significant mediators in the relationship between self-concept and academic achievement (Khalaila, 2015).

---

## ▦ SUMMARY

Academia promotes an atmosphere that influences educators to challenge themselves to exceed standard expectations. Making the decision to take the CNEcl certification examination allows clinical nurse educators to validate their expertise and knowledge through certification. Certification tests are intimidating for essentially every examination candidate. Regardless of your reason for wanting to obtain this certification, a critical step is familiarizing yourself with the basics of test design and concepts. Candidates who pass the examination can use the CNEcl certification following their names as long as the certification remains valid. Certification is valid for 5 years. Clinical nurse educators who are certified are invaluable resources who serve as mentors, role models, and visionaries. They are crucial in assisting future nurse educators and enhancing the teaching–learning process by advancing academic standards within the discipline.

### 2.1 Case Study

The clinical nurse educator is in the CLE assisting one of the learners to administer medications. Another learner from the same clinical group is extremely excited and comes up to the clinical nurse educator and states that the primary nurse allowed her to administer furosemide 40 mg IV (intravenous) push. The learner emphasized that the primary nurse was present the entire time the medication was being given. The clinical nurse educator is aware that the educational institution in which she is employed does not permit learners to give medications using this route. However, the clinical institution does have a policy allowing learners to carry out this procedure. There were no untoward effects from the patient who received the medication.

**Questions for Reflection:**

1. Which policy should the clinical nurse educator follow?
2. What actions should the clinical nurse educator take to address this incident?

CLE, clinical learning environment.

### 2.2 Case Study

During postconference, one of the learners asks you specific questions that were on an exam the class recently had taken. The learner feels the course faculty has made an error when filling in the answer key. This conversation gains the interest of the other learners in the group and they are now requesting your input.

**Questions for Reflection:**

1. Should the clinical nurse educator discuss this issue with the learners to verify whether their statements are accurate?
2. What is the best approach that should be taken by the clinical nurse educator?

## ▦ REVIEW QUESTIONS

1. The clinical nurse educator observed that students were struggling with normal lab values. She creates an electronic Jeopardy game using brief scenarios to enhance their knowledge base. This teaching strategy would be most effective for which type of learner?

   A. Visual

   B. Auditory

   C. Kinesthetic

   D. Read/Write

2. The examination candidate should make which content area a priority as it accounts for 19% of the exam items.

   A. Facilitate Learning in the Healthcare Environment

   B. Facilitate Learner Development and Socialization

   C. Implement Effective Clinical Assessment and Evaluation Strategies

   D. Apply Clinical Expertise in the Healthcare Environment

3. On the day of the examination, which would be the most nutritious food choice for the candidate to consume?

   A. Bran muffin and a soy latte with two shots of expresso

   B. Two chocolate eclairs with a glass of whole milk

   C. Whole wheat bagel and a fruit smoothie with kale

   D. Cheese omelette with an orange energy drink

4. Which of the following is an example of surface learning?

   A. Making links between concepts

   B. Memorizing facts, figures, and tables

   C. Relating current material to previously learned material

   D. Organizing information into categories

5. After a simulation experience, the clinical nurse educator conducts a debriefing session. According to Bloom's taxonomy, which domain of behavior is being evaluated?

   A. Cognitive

   B. Affective

   C. Psychomotor

   D. Comprehension

6. The clinical nurse educator develops a case study for the students to complete during a postconference. One of the requirements is for the student to create a teaching plan for the patient. Which of the following cognitive levels is being asked of the student?

   A. Knowledge

   B. Application

   C. Analysis

   D. Synthesis

7. Which of the following demonstrates an effective method of studying?

   A. Answering practice questions that mimic the actual certification exam, including environment and time frame

   B. Identifying the tricks and strategies of the examination to reduce the amount of material that needs to be studied

   C. Read only the rationales to questions you answered incorrectly while taking practice exams

   D. Study only when time allows within your schedule

8. Which eligibility criteria must be met to sit for the Certified Academic Clinical Nurse Educator (CNEcl) certification examination and is found in both options?

   A. A baccalaureate degree in nursing

   B. Two years of teaching experience in an academic setting within the least 5 years

   C. A graduate degree with a focus on nursing education

   D. Three years in any area of nursing practice

9. A candidate fails her certification exam the first time she sits for it. She asks whether she can reapply to retake the exam. What is the best response to provide to her?

   A. "No, since you have taken it and were unsuccessful, there is no chance to retake the test."

   B. "Yes, you can retake the exam but you must sit for a remediation course before you can reapply."

   C. "Yes, you can retake the exam in 90 days but cannot exceed taking the exam four times within a year."

   D. "No, because you have seen the questions on the exam and it would not be a fair assessment of your actual performance."

10. A clinical nurse educator, who took and passed the exam 6 years ago, continues to use the credential "Certified Academic Clinical Nurse Educator (CNEcl)" after her name. When asked whether she has renewed her certification, she denies doing so. What would be the best response by the director of the nursing program in which she is employed?

    A. "You can continue to use those credentials; however, please renew this certification as soon as possible."

    B. "You are not permitted to use those credentials any longer since it is only valid for 5 years and you must retake the examination since you allowed the certification to expire."

    C. "It is fortunate for you that one does not have to renew this certification."

    D. "Since you are currently in a teaching position and you are assigned to clinical with students, recertification is not required."

## ▪ REFERENCES

Blevins, S. (2014). Understanding learning styles. *MedSurg Nursing, 23*(1), 59–60.

Chan, Z. C. Y. (2017). A qualitative study on using concept maps in problem-based learning. *Nurse Education in Practice, 24,* 70–76.

Fleming, N. (2001). *Teaching and learning styles: VARK strategies.* Christchurch, NZ: Author.

Fressola, M. C., & Patterson, G. E. (2017). *Transition from clinician to educator: A practical approach.* Burlington, MA: Jones & Bartlett Learning.

Institute of Medicine. (2010). *The future of nursing: Leading change, advancing health.* Washington, DC: National Academies Press. Retrieved from http://www.nationalacademies.org/hmd/Reports/2010/The-Future-of-Nursing-Leading- Change-Advancing-Health.aspx

Khalaila, R. (2015). The relationship between academic self-concept, intrinsic motivation, test anxiety, and academic achievement among nursing students: Mediating and moderating effects. *Nurse Education Today, 35,* 432–438. doi:10.1016/j.nedt.2014.11.001

Lovecchio, C., DiMattio, M. J. K., & Hudacek, S. (2015). Predictors of undergraduate nursing student satisfaction with clinical learning environment: A secondary analysis. *Nursing Education Perspectives, 30,* 274–279. doi:10.5480/13-1266

McDonald, M. E. (2018). *The nurse educator's guide to assessing learning outcomes.* Burlington, MA: Jones & Bartlett Learning.

National League for Nursing. (2018). *Certified Academic Clinical Nurse Educator (CNE®cl) 2018 candidate handbook.* Retrieved from http://www.nln.org/docs/default-source/default-document-library/CNE®cl-handbook-jan-2018.pdf?sfvrsn=4

Sawchuk, C. N. (2017). *Is it possible to overcome test anxiety?* Retrieved from https://www.mayoclinic.org/diseases-conditions/generalized-anxiety-disorder/expert-answers/test-anxiety/faq-20058195

Shushan, J. H. (2017). *A pocket guide to college success* (2nd ed.). Boston, MA: Macmillan Learning.

U.S. Bureau of Labor Statistics. (2018). *Occupational outlook handbook.* Retrieved from https://www.bls.gov/ooh/healthcare

VARK®. (n.d). *VARK®: A guide to learning preferences.* Retrieved from http://vark-learn.com/

Wilson, L., & Wittmann-Price, R. A. (2015). *Certified healthcare simulation educator (CHSE™) exam.* New York. NY: Springer Publishing Company,.

Wittmann-Price, R. A., Godshall, M., & Wilson, L. (2017). *Certified nurse educator (CNE) review manual* (3rd ed.). New York, NY: Springer Publishing Company.

# 3 Functioning Within the Education and Healthcare Environments: Function in the Clinical Educator Role

*KAREN K. GITTINGS*

> *Better than a thousand days of diligent study is one day with a great teacher.*
> —Japanese Proverb

## ■ LEARNING OUTCOMES

At the end of this chapter, the learner will be able to

1. Appraise strategies that can be employed to bridge the gap between theory and practice.
2. Examine techniques that guide the development of professional behaviors.
3. Identify technological advances useful for learning in the clinical learning environment (CLE).
4. Evaluate the influence of role models in the development of professional behaviors.
5. Determine the importance of inclusive excellence in the CLE.

## ■ INTRODUCTION

Clinical nurse educators are in a unique situation in that they must be able to function competently as an academic in the educational environment and as a practice nurse in the healthcare environment. The challenging role of the clinical nurse educator melds together the worlds of education and practice. Although the educator often has extensive nursing practice experience, many lack formal education in teaching.

There are many roles that the clinical nurse educator must learn in order to be effective, including bridging the gap between theory and practice, fostering professional growth in learners, using technologies to enhance teaching and learning, valuing the contributions of others, acting as a role model, and demonstrating inclusive excellence. This chapter describes recommendations for operationalizing the role of the clinical nurse educator.

## BRIDGING THE GAP BETWEEN THEORY AND PRACTICE

A significant challenge that nursing students face is bridging the theory–practice gap. In the classroom setting, students are taught theoretical information, which must in turn be translated into usable information in the practice environment. Academic nurse educators strive to make information relatable and applicable to clinical practice, but it is the clinical nurse educator who is at the point of contact and must be relied upon to assist students to make these vital connections.

Nursing programs have hundreds of required clinical hours, yet a review of the literature documents that a gap commonly occurs between theory and practice among graduate nurses. With the current shortage of RNs in the United States, clinical agencies need newly hired RNs to acclimate quickly and to demonstrate competence in the practice setting. Unfortunately, new graduates are having difficulty making the transition to practice. This makes it incumbent upon nursing programs to better prepare students to bridge the theory–practice gap. The clinical practice environment for student nurses is becoming increasingly important and the role of the clinical nurse educator is vital to their success.

Clinical nurse educators are needed to facilitate the development of clinical skills and the application of knowledge to practice for nursing students. Clinical nurse educators are also challenged to assist students with the development of clinical decision-making skills. Along with decision-making skills, students need to be socialized into the role of the professional nurse (Patterson, Boyd, & Mnatzaganian, 2017). Perhaps the most challenging of these skills to teach is that of clinical decision-making when it pertains to real-life patient situations.

The *theory of cognitive apprenticeship* was developed in response to the recognized theory–practice gap. *Cognitive apprenticeship* is described by Collins (as cited in Lyons, McLaughlin, Khanova, & Roth, 2017, p. 724) as "making expert thinking 'visible' to the learner." This process is akin to the apprenticeship model except instead of the learner observing physical skills, she or he is observing cognitive processes. Through cognitive apprenticeship, learners are able to better develop clinical decision-making skills.

Lyons et al. (2017) describe the following methods as useful in cognitive apprenticeship:

- Modeling
- Coaching
- Scaffolding
- Articulation
- Reflection
- Exploration

The clinical nurse educator can use these methods to assist learners to develop clinical decision-making skills. In modeling, the clinical nurse educator can demonstrate skills, behaviors, or attributes. As coach, the clinical nurse educator observes a student demonstration and provides individualized feedback. With scaffolding, the clinical nurse educator provides support, hints, and reminders. Using articulation, students are required to explain their rationales for decisions. The clinical nurse educator can encourage reflection through discussions or journals. Finally, using exploration, the clinical nurse educator stimulates the learner to ask more questions and to apply their new knowledge and skills (Lyons et al., 2017).

Although cognitive apprenticeship has been found effective in clinical instruction, Lyons et al. (2017) recommend formal training for clinical nurse educators in order for the experience to be effective and meaningful. Nursing programs that utilize cognitive apprenticeship should invest in the education of the clinical nurse educators so that the method is effective. The goal in incorporating the cognitive apprenticeship model and its intendant methods is to improve clinical decision-making as students traverse the theory–practice gap.

Students face many sources of stress and anxiety in the CLE, including the unpredictability of the environment and increased patient acuity, attitudes of the professional nursing and ancillary staff, interactions with multiple professionals, and the disconnect between textbook information and that which is learned in the classroom and the "real world" (Patterson et al., 2017). The clinical nurse educator is challenged to promote an environment that is conducive to reducing student stress and encouraging learning.

The traditional clinical model used by many nursing programs in the United States is not always successful in achieving environments that are conducive to student learning. In a study by Patterson et al. (2017), the authors found that students who participated in a university fellowship program (UFP) that focused their clinical experiences in one single organization, resulted in graduates who were more work ready than graduates who were educated using other clinical models. Although the UFP is not widely utilized in the United States, this study illustrates the importance of collaboration between the nursing program and the healthcare organization. As the clinical nurse educator strives to promote an effective learning environment, it is vital that a professional, conciliatory relationship be developed. A collaborative relationship is one in which the clinical nurse educator, professional nursing staff, and healthcare team can work together in promoting an environment conducive to learning.

To further promote an environment conducive to learning, the clinical nurse educator must utilize effective teaching and learning strategies that match the needs of the learners. Specifically, the clinical nurse educator should consider the following:

- Motivation for learning
- Student attributes
- Application of effective clinical teaching strategies (Battle & Tyson, 2018)

Although nontraditional students are increasing in number, the majority of students are still the traditional 18- to 24-year-olds. Fortunately, as adult learners, traditional and nontraditional students are often motivated to succeed. This motivation can come from either *extrinsic or intrinsic factors*. A student who is extrinsically motivated will be influenced by the environment, whereas a student who is intrinsically motivated will perform in response to internal needs and desires (Battle & Tyson, 2018). The clinical nurse educator uses this knowledge when dealing with individual students. For example, the extrinsically motivated student may act based on a desire to achieve high grades. The intrinsically motivated student may respond better to positive feedback and a sense of accomplishment. The clinical nurse educator who develops an understanding of his or her students' motivation is better able to meet student learning needs in the CLE.

It is also important for the clinical nurse educator to understand *generational differences* in learners. Currently, learners can be classified into three groups, including the baby boomers (born between 1945 and 1960), generation X (1960–1980), and the millennials (1980–2000). The way in which these groups best learn is affected by historical events, cultural influences, and societal values that occurred as they grew to adulthood (Battle & Tyson, 2018). The clinical nurse educator should take into consideration generational attributes when planning teaching and learning activities. For example,

- The baby boomer, who has great respect for authority, best learns when the focus is teacher-directed.
- Learners who are generation Xers are more independent and creative; they learn better with learner-directed activities.
- The millennials, who comprise a large number of today's students, are confident, team-oriented, and technologically savvy. These learners prefer the use of technology, collaboration, and immediate feedback (Battle & Tyson, 2018).

The challenge for the clinical nurse educator is to be flexible in using teaching and learning strategies in the CLE to provide optimal learning opportunities for all students.

To provide the best environment for learning, in addition to taking into consideration the student's motivation to learn and generational attributes, the clinical nurse educator should also utilize a variety of instructional methods to reach a majority of the learners. Interactive strategies that engage the learner are particularly important in the CLE as learners are assisted in translating theory to practice and developing clinical competence.

Active learning strategies are important for developing critical thinking and clinical decision-making skills. Although active learning can be effective for all students, millennials, in particular, respond well to this strategy. Examples of active learning opportunities in the CLE include the following:

- Simulation

- Service learning

- Internships and/or preceptorships (Battle & Tyson, 2018)

*Simulation* provides an opportunity to practice skills in a nonthreatening environment as well as to practice skills that are not readily available in the CLE. With high-fidelity simulation, students are able to apply knowledge and further develop critical thinking skills. The National League for Nursing (as cited in Battle & Tyson, 2018) identifies *simulation* as an experiential learning opportunity in which learners develop clinical decision-making skills that further facilitate transition to practice. Clinical nurse educators often have assigned responsibilities as their students participate in simulation activities. It is imperative that clinical nurse educators understand the desired outcomes for the simulation so that they can effectively interact with learners and answer questions that may occur during the simulation or in the CLE following the experience (additional simulation information is provided in Chapter 4, Functioning Within the Education and Healthcare Environments: Operationalize the Curriculum).

*Service learning* provides learners with the opportunity to apply what they have learned in the real world (Battle & Tyson, 2018). Although traditional clinical experiences are not usually referred to as *service learning*, they can be categorized as such. Clinical nurse educators who are working in the acute care setting typically have direct oversight of their students. When service learning occurs in the community setting, clinical nurse educators may have more of an indirect influence because students are usually in multiple locations assigned to professional nursing staff.

In *internships* or *preceptorships*, learners usually work directly under the supervision of an RN employed by the facility (Battle & Tyson, 2018). In such cases, the clinical nurse educator typically has more of an oversight role with less direct contact. In these settings, the professional nursing staff typically has more of an influence than the clinical nurse educator. Students have the opportunity to apply theory to practice as they work one-on-one with an assigned RN. The clinical nurse educator's role is to ensure that the environment is conducive to student learning.

The active learning strategies of simulation, service learning, and internships/preceptorships are effective methods in promoting clinical decision-making skills as students work to overcome the theory–practice gap. The role of the clinical nurse educator can vary depending on the strategy used, ranging from direct oversight to indirect supervision. Whatever the clinical nurse educator's role, it is most important that the CLE is conducive to learning to best prepare students to transition to practice.

Even with best laid plans, not all clinical experiences are successful in promoting student learning. Multiple factors can influence the effectiveness of the CLE, including the following:

- Instructor/educator
- Students
- Professional nursing staff and healthcare professionals
- Physical environment

If any combination of these factors are insufficient, student learning may be impacted. In a study by Gunay and Kilinc (2018), the authors interviewed nursing students to better understand their clinical experiences. Almost half of the students identified difficulties in the CLE with the most important being the inability to put theoretical information into practice. Students also identified that skills learned in the laboratory setting are not always practiced in the same way in the CLE. This provides further evidence that students have difficulty bridging the theory–practice gap.

Other themes identified by Gunay and Kilinc (2018) included the following:

- Lack of sufficient support from the clinical nurse educator
- Lack of support from professional nursing staff
- Lack of opportunities to practice skills
- Limitations with the physical environment

Based on these findings, the important role that the clinical nurse educator has in facilitating a successful clinical experience is evident. It is important for the clinical nurse educator to be a knowledgeable and skillful practitioner. In addition, the educator should be "approachable, supportive, helpful, empathetic, and encouraging" (Gunay & Kilinc, 2018, p. 85). The educator needs to be attuned to the attitudes and behaviors of professional nursing staff. Although most nurses are supportive of students, there are still those who view students as being in the way and time-consuming. The nurse educator is in a position to promote collaboration as well as facilitate communication between the professional nursing staff and students. As an advocate for the learners, the clinical nurse educator may need to intervene in situations that detract from the learning experience.

Throughout the clinical experience, the clinical nurse educator should evaluate the physical environment to ensure it is conducive to student learning. Are there sufficient opportunities for students to practice skills? Is there a sufficient number of patients for the number of students on the unit? Are there enough computers for the students to review patient records, administer medications, and/or document care? Is there a location where students can take a break and store their personal belongings? The physical environment must also be conducive to student learning.

---

**3.1  Clinical Nurse Educator Teaching Tip**

Clinical nurse educators tend to overlook the importance of the physical environment because they may believe they have no input there. Many programs have students as well as the clinical nurse educators evaluate the CLE to determine its effectiveness in helping students achieve the SLOs. Even if a program does not have a formal evaluation process, it is important that clinical nurse educators keep course faculty apprised of any issues so that only CLEs that are conducive to learning are used.

CLE, clinical learning environment; SLOs, student learning outcomes.

---

The clinical nurse educator has a significant role in promoting an effective CLE. For students to develop clinical decision-making skills, the CLE must:

- Present the opportunity for skills attainment, problem-solving, and critical thinking.
- Promote effective communication and collaboration among the clinical nurse educator, students, and professional nursing staff.

In providing a CLE that encourages and allows for growth, the clinical nurse educator is providing the student with the best opportunity to bridge the theory–practice gap.

## ▓ FOSTERING PROFESSIONAL GROWTH

An important role of the clinical nurse educator is to assist learners to grow in competence as they progress through a nursing curriculum. Ideally, learners should develop knowledge, skills, and attitudes that will prepare them for practice as novice graduate nurses. Clinical decision-making, or clinical judgment, is an important skill to be learned. Tanner (as cited in AL Sabei & Lasater, 2016) defines *clinical judgment* as "an interpretation or conclusion about a patient's needs, concerns, or health problems, and/or the decision to take action (or not), use or modify standard approaches, or improvise new ones as deemed appropriate by the patient's response" (p. 42). It is the clinical nurse educator who prepares learners to function safely and competently in the CLE. In fostering professional growth in learners, the clinical nurse educator often uses the techniques of coaching, reflection, and debriefing.

In order to make appropriate clinical decisions, Tanner (as cited in AL Sabei & Lasater, 2016) describes the reflective processes of *reflection-in-action* and *reflection-on-action*. *Reflection-in-action* refers to the interpretation of the patient's condition, interventions used, the patient's response, and the nurse's reassessment and continued interventions in response to the patient's ongoing situation. *Reflection-on-action* refers to the nurse's evaluation of lessons learned from the event and future applications of the learning. AL Sabei and Lasater propose a definition of *debriefing* based on Tanner's work, "a structured and guided reflection process through which students actively appraise their cognitive, affective, and psychomotor performance within the context of their clinical judgment skill" (p. 43). *Debriefing* has three important qualities:

- Reflection offers a time to review and analyze one's performance
- Learners are actively engaged through questioning
- Facilitators can assist learners to apply theory to practice

Debriefing has been widely discussed in the literature concerning simulation, but it is also relevant for use in the CLE. In a review of the literature, Dufrene and Young (2014) found debriefing, no matter the strategy used, to be effective in improving learner performance. Reflection is an important aspect of debriefing that facilitates the learner's understanding of the cause, action, and consequences in a given situation. This can result in improved surveillance skills and knowledge of how to act in similar situations (Lavoie, Pepin, & Cossette, 2017). Using *reflective debriefing*, the clinical nurse educator can assist the learner to connect the events of the patient situation to the outcomes of her or his actions. In this manner, students can learn how to respond appropriately in future situations. It is incumbent upon the clinical nurse educator to encourage active student participation during the debriefing while providing constructive feedback. In addition, clinical nurse educators must ask questions that elicit higher ordered thinking. For novice educators, it is helpful to have a structured debriefing format for guidance (AL Sabei & Lasater, 2016).

Clinical decision-making, which is often lacking in new graduates, can be improved through the use of debriefing. Dreifuerst (as cited in Forneris et al., 2015) developed the Debriefing for Meaningful Learning (DML) method, which has been found to positively impact clinical reasoning. The DML is a structured process of reflection and dialogue in which learners are guided to analyze their action; this knowledge acquisition can be applied in future practice situations. In a study by Forneris et al., nursing students who were debriefed using the DML method were found to have higher clinical reasoning scores when compared to students who were debriefed through customary means. In using the DML method, the clinical nurse educator is able to guide students through reflection and discussion on a clinical scenario and role-model her or his own thought process in arriving at a solution.

Kuiper et al. (as cited in Forneris et al., 2015) developed the Outcome–Present State Test (OPT) model and worksheet, which is another method for structured debriefing. This method also incorporates reflection, which can be utilized in clinical practice as well as simulation. The clinical nurse educator is able to utilize the OPT model to encourage the learner to think about the reason behind her or his actions.

Debriefing is traditionally done by a nurse educator, in some cases, the clinical nurse educator. No matter who facilitates the experience, it is more important that the person performing the debriefing be adequately trained in the process. In a study by Kang and Yu (2018), it was found that student self-debriefing (SSD) combined with instructor-led debriefing (ID) resulted in higher problem-solving scores and debriefing satisfaction when compared to ID alone. The clinical nurse educator may consider including student self-debriefing, but in order to correct any inaccuracies, instructor-led feedback is also needed.

The clinical nurse educator may utilize debriefing following a scenario in the simulation laboratory or following a patient event in the CLE. This active teaching–learning strategy has been found effective in assisting students to transfer new knowledge to future situations and in developing clinical decision-making skills (Forneris et al., 2015). For learning to occur, there must be a discussion, analysis, and summarization following the simulation and/or patient event. The clinical nurse educator facilitates a discussion of the event, provides time for reflection, and assists learners to understand the consequences of their actions (Kang & Yu, 2018). The International Nursing Association for Clinical Simulation and Learning (as cited in Kang & Yu, 2018) has identified the importance of the facilitator being trained in the debriefing process. It is therefore important that the clinical nurse educator be trained and prepared in order to provide effective debriefing, whether in the simulation or CLE.

---

**3.1 Evidence-Based Clinical Teaching Practice**

In a study by Gantt, Overton, Avery, Swanson, and Elhammoumi (2018), undergraduate nursing students were divided into four groups to determine the most effective method for debriefing. The first group received facilitated debriefing whereby faculty led a full discussion of the events. In the second group, self-debriefing was done with a tool using the plus/delta method. Feedback was used with the third group, in which important actions were identified, but no discussion occurred. The fourth group served as the control. Results

(continued)

| 3.1   Evidence-Based Clinical Teaching Practice (*continued*) |
| --- |
| showed that the facilitated debriefing group had significantly greater scores in follow-up simulations. Overall, students and faculty also expressed a preference for the facilitated debriefing. |

In addition to the need for nursing students to develop clinical decision-making skills and competence, it is likewise important to prepare these students for their *professional nursing role*. Clinical nurse educators play a vital role in socializing learners to the personal and professional expectations of nursing. Reflective journals are a teaching–learning strategy that facilitates the development of professional, cognitive, and affective attributes. A study by Mahlanze and Sibiya (2017) described the effects of reflective journaling on the personal development and clinical learning of undergraduate nursing students. Findings include the following:

- Improved problem-solving

- Improved self-awareness

- Improved response to variable situations

In using reflective journaling, the clinical nurse educator must allow sufficient time for reflection, as change occurs over time. The educator must also clearly explain the purpose, process, and benefits of reflective journaling so that students put forth their best effort in engaging in self-reflection. A trusting relationship between the educator and student is necessary for the learner to feel safe in sharing personal feelings. The clinical nurse educator must cautiously provide feedback that is non-judgmental for learners to feel safe in expressing themselves (Mahlanze & Sibiya, 2017).

Today's graduate nurses also need to be prepared to function as leaders in an increasingly complex healthcare environment. The clinical nurse educator should plan assignments that promote managerial and *leadership skills*. An assignment that provides the opportunity to function in the role of the nurse, including decision-making opportunities, is more effective than observational experiences. Providing opportunities for delegation and teamwork facilitates the use of leadership skills. In a study of nursing students' experiences with clinical leadership, Demeh and Rosengren (2015) found that exposure to managerial and leadership opportunities facilitate the transition to practice. Nursing students identified the importance of clinical nurse educators acting as a resource in preparing them for the role of the nurse. The clinical nurse educator role-models effective, constructive communication skills necessary for clinical leadership. Coaching is also effective in promoting personal growth and professional development in nursing students (Demeh & Rosengren, 2015). In a review of the literature by Walker, Cooke, Henderson, and Creedy (2011), it was identified that the clinical nurse manager is vital in promoting an environment conducive to learning and positive nursing role models are linked to supportive learning environments. This additionally supports the importance of positive role-modeling behaviors by the clinical nurse educator. The clinical nurse educator, nurse manager, and professional nursing staff all play an important role in fostering the professional growth of nursing students.

## ■ USING TECHNOLOGY

*Technological advances* and usage in the CLE are only going to increase in the coming years. The clinical nurse educator will need to ensure that students are able to function in this technologically rich environment and, in some cases, lead the way in making changes. It is ironic that in many situations, it is the students who are more technologically savvy than the educators. The challenge then is for these educators to improve their comfort with and knowledge of technology so that they can be a resource for their students.

The National League for Nursing (as cited in Risling, 2017, p. 89) has issued a call for action that highlights the need for nursing programs to "teach with and about technology." Because legislation has mandated the use of electronic health records (EHRs), clinical nurse educators and students must be able to function using these systems to provide patient care, as well as have sufficient knowledge to educate patients on the use of patient EHR portals. Clinical nurse educators must prepare learners to work with the evolving development of monitoring systems. In addition, educators must assist learners to identify reliable sites on the Internet to be used to educate patients about accurate information retrieval (Risling, 2017).

Mobile devices, such as smartphones and tablets, are being increasingly utilized in the CLE. Instead of relying on the recall of information taught in the classroom setting, learners are now able to construct their own knowledge using information available through mobile technology. Multiple uses have been identified for mobile technology in the CLE, including retrieval of information pertaining to medications and laboratory results and access to evidence-based resources or decision aids. Mackay, Anderson, and Harding (2017) identified enabling and constraining factors that influence the use of mobile devices in the CLE. Factors that enable and/or encourage the clinical nurse educator to utilize mobile technology include the following:

- Immediate access to a multitude of resources
- Promotion of evidence-based practice with easy access to references
- Access to enhanced teaching applications that can be used in the CLE
- Active engagement of learners of all types
- Facilitation of communication with colleagues and/or students while in the CLE

- Start-up and ongoing information technology (IT) support

Factors that may inhibit the use of mobile technology by the clinical nurse educator include the following:

- Perceptions (of educator and/or professional nursing staff) that using a device in the CLE is unprofessional
- Lack of knowledge and skill in using technology
- Connectivity issues
- Policies prohibiting usage

In order to utilize technology to its fullest extent and capability, the clinical nurse educator must strive to minimize those factors that deter its use. The educator who questions the professionalism of using mobile devices in the CLE should first examine his or her own motives and beliefs related to use of these devices. It is also helpful to consider the benefits and drawbacks of utilizing mobile technology in this setting. When professional nursing staff are resistant to the use of mobile technology, the clinical nurse educator can serve as a role model for professional use. Educators can also seek to be a part of policy development related to the use of mobile devices in the CLE. Finally, for those clinical nurse educators who are not as technologically savvy, IT and course faculty support are essential in providing necessary training, updates, and continuing education to increase the comfort level of those who are less technologically inclined. Fiedler, Giddens, and North (2014) have identified the importance of institutional support when adopting new technologies. Clinical nurse educators can become discouraged if they perceive that they have not been adequately trained or lack sufficient support. Educators need time to learn the new technology and feel confident in its use so that they in turn can be a resource to students adopting the new technology.

For all the noted advantages of mobile technology, there have been concerns that use of these devices can be distracting for the healthcare provider. To be specific, Porter (as cited in Cho & Lee, 2016) found that smartphone usage could prolong response times, minimize attention, and alter the caregiver's performance overall, resulting in potential patient safety issues. There is an additional concern that use of social media is increasing during work hours. The Emergency Care Research Institute (as cited in Cho & Lee, 2016) in 2013 found that distractions from mobile devices were the ninth highest health technology hazard. In their study of nursing students, Cho and Lee (2016) found that 46.2% used smartphones in the CLE. A low number of students (27.9%) reported being distracted by smartphone use, but 42.9% noticed others being distracted. In response to these concerns, organizations are instituting policies that prohibit, limit, or strongly regulate the use of mobile technology, particularly smartphone use. The clinical nurse educator is responsible for ensuring that learners adhere to organizational polices related to the use of smartphones and other mobile technology. The clinical nurse educator must also provide education and monitoring related to appropriate usage and the potential for distraction related to patient care and safety.

Perceptions also play a role in the use of mobile technology. A study by McNally, Frey, and Crossan (2017) compared the perceptions of nurse managers and student nurses on the use of mobile devices in the CLE. Nurse managers, although in favor of the accessibility of smartphones to resources used to improve patient care, viewed use of these devices overall as unprofessional. There was also a lack of trust that students were using the devices appropriately and not spending time on social media. Students expressed concern that the nurses and manager might view them as unprofessional for using this technology, but they also identified the many positives aspects of mobile technology, including access to multiple resources and references that can assist with patient care. McNally et al. also identified that students often lack education on the identification of reliable applications and Internet sites. Roberts and Williams (2017) identified the usefulness of mobile technology in the CLE when computers are not always abundant and available for student use or when access to the Internet is blocked; however, the greatest difficulty for learners is in discerning credible sources.

The clinical nurse educator needs to be acutely aware of the clinical nursing environment. In settings where mobile technology is viewed negatively, the clinical nurse educator could use the opportunity to educate the professional nursing staff and/or manager about the advantages of these devices. It is also important that the educator and students model acceptable uses of their devices and to avoid even the appearance of distraction and/or isolation. The clinical nurse educator must be clear that social networking in the CLE is prohibited. The educator can act as a resource in assisting learners to identify credible resources. Providing learners with information on how to evaluate informational sites and/or a list of popular, valid resources would be helpful. The educator should also check in with the course faculty to determine whether any electronic book resources were required for the course, for example, medication resources.

With the growth of technology, nursing programs may need to consider the addition of informatics courses to provide necessary education; however, whether a program has an informatics course or not, it will fall to the clinical nurse educator to ensure that students are able to safely utilize technology in the CLE. Instruction related to legal and ethical issues must also be provided. With the increased use use of smartphones and social networking, the clinical nurse educator must encourage professional behavior and warn students of the risk for breaches in privacy and confidentiality these pose.

## ▪ VALUING THE CONTRIBUTIONS OF OTHERS

Clinical nurse educators should recognize that students often face barriers to successful completion of the nursing program. The most commonly cited issues include the following:

- Finances

- Academic performance

- Time management

- Family obligations

- Pace of the program (Dewitty, Huerta, & Downing, 2016)

The clinical nurse educator is generally unable to provide assistance with financial and family issues, but may be able to offer helpful suggestions with time-management and academic concerns. Because many clinical nurse educators are part-time faculty, they may lack information on all the resources available, so communication with the course faculty is imperative. In assisting students to learn and deal with barriers as they arise, the educator needs to recognize that there are often many people who contribute to the students' success.

People who influence and contribute to students' success include families, mentors, role models, and/or faculty (Dewitty et al., 2016). Although families can serve as a barrier at times because of demands placed on the student's time, for the most part, families are a valuable support system and play a significant role in the student's success. Students may need guidance to maneuver through family and school obligations. Clinical nurse educators, while recognizing the importance of family, may be able to offer additional suggestions about effective time management.

Mentors can assist with professional and career guidance. Most undergraduate nursing students will not have a mentor unless one is assigned. Some nursing programs utilize mentoring partnerships with peers (higher level nursing students), faculty, or alumni. For students seeking a mentor, the clinical nurse educator may have contacts that would be willing to assist. The support and advice provided by mentors can be extremely helpful to the student trying to progress through the nursing program and into that first entry-level job.

Role models also contribute to the students' development of professional attitudes and behaviors. In the CLE, students are watching all that is happening around them. The professional nursing staff can be very influential as students learn professionalism and how to conduct themselves as nurses. The clinical nurse educator often serves as a role model for students, but she or he must also be aware that students will also choose to role-model behaviors of others, particularly the professional nursing staff. The educator should see the value in what role models can teach, but be wary of those who might demonstrate poor behaviors that should not be adopted.

The clinical nurse educator is perhaps the most important contributor to students' success in the CLE, but it is important for educators to remember that they are not alone. The professional nursing staff, mentors, those who serve as role models, and families all play a part in contributing to the students' success. When the clinical nurse educator recognizes, values, and utilizes all available resources, the chances of student success are magnified.

## ▨ ACTING AS ROLE MODEL

In assisting students to develop into competent graduate nurses who can adapt to the practice setting, the clinical nurse educator plays a vital part in role-modeling the attributes of a professional nurse. Although the act of role-modeling is often unconscious, the educator must be cognizant that students are watching at all times. The clinical nurse educator must ensure that professional behavior is always being exhibited to avoid role-modeling poor behaviors.

Role-modeling has been described by Cruess (as cited in Baldwin, Mills, Birks, & Budden, 2014) as the adoption of attitudes and/or behaviors exhibited by one who is admired. In a review of the literature, Baldwin et al. reviewed studies done pertaining to nurse clinicians (including clinical nurse educators) and nurse academics as role models. In studies that focused on the effect of nurse clinicians as role models, learners were found to mimic those they viewed as being good nurses, but it was additionally noted that even those viewed as poor nurses had a beneficial effect in that students made a conscious decision to not emulate those attitudes and/or behaviors perceived as inappropriate. Nurses identified as good role models demonstrated characteristics such as respect for students, excellence in patient care, and incorporation of evidence-based guidelines into patient care. Additional traits identified included the following:

- Approachable
- Ability to instill confidence
- Available
- Student advocate
- Tolerates student mistakes
- Demonstrates respect for students
- Provides timely feedback (Baldwin et al., 2014, p. e24)

Studies done on the effect of nursing academics as role models have identified similar traits. Enthusiasm and positive attitudes toward nursing were additionally found to be important characteristics. It is important to note that students will quickly gauge a clinical nurse educator as being a good or bad role model.

A vital piece to bridging the theory–practice gap is assisting learners to develop critical thinking. Clinical nurse educators play an integral part in the development of clinical decision-making skills. Raymond,

Profetto-McGrath, Myrick, and Strean (2018) studied clinical nurse educators to determine how they role-model critical thinking in the CLE. The results were divided into the categories of questioning, personal dispositions, and teaching. Characteristics that relate to questioning include the following:

- Uses variable question levels.
- Asks "why" questions.
- Follows up with students.
- Encourages curiosity.

Characteristics that relate to personal dispositions include the following:

- Humble about personal knowledge and deficits
- Approachable
- Embraces diversity
- Sense of curiosity
- Flexible

Characteristics that relate to teaching include the following:

- Thinks out loud.
- Practices quality care.
- Utilizes resources.
- Encourages collaborative problem-solving (Raymond et al., 2018)

The study by Raymond et al. (2018) demonstrates how role-modeling can be used in teaching critical thinking. Clinical nurse educators should consider the adoption of these traits in guiding students to make good clinical decisions. Educators often ask themselves how they can teach their students to think critically and make good decisions. One approach is to encourage a CLE in which students are encouraged to question and where mistakes are viewed as learning opportunities. A clinical nurse educator who demonstrates excellence in patient care and allows the student to see her or his thinking is providing an opportunity to observe clinical decision-making through role-modeling.

Students in the CLE may also look to professional nursing staff as role models. Bandura (as cited in Felstead & Springett, 2016) noted that people are more likely to adopt behaviors if they result in outcomes the individuals value and lead to positive consequences; however, Henderson (as cited in Felstead & Springett, 2016) also found that students may mimic poor practice if this is common in the CLE and students believe that they need to adapt for learning to be successful. In their own study, Felstead and Springett (2016) found that staff nurses are often looked upon as role models who significantly influence students' development. Leading by example was considered an important characteristic. Students also identified the importance of strong, effective leadership and indicated that weak leadership could lead to problems with communication, teamwork, and morale. Although this study focused on the professional nursing staff as role models, it is important that the clinical nurse educator understand the influence she or he holds over students.

The clinical nurse educator needs to have an awareness of the professional nursing staff working with the learners in the CLE. Knowing that students are always observing and can feel pressure to conform, it is important that the clinical nurse educator address attitudes and behaviors that are unprofessional and/or unsafe. This may be as simple as speaking with a nurse to remind the nurse that students are malleable and need to learn best practice, but it may need to go further if unprofessional behaviors continue. The clinical nurse educator may need to address issues with the nurse manager or with students in postconference. In the extreme, the clinical nurse educator may need to avoid assigning students to work with certain nurses. Ideally, students should have the opportunity to learn from the best role models, whether these are clinical nurse educators or professional nursing staff.

The influence that clinical nurse educators have on learners cannot be understated. In order for educators to be viewed as positive role models, it is important that they have guidance and support from the course faculty and other educational resource people. Clinical nurse educators should also take advantage of professional development and continuing-education opportunities so they are informed on best practices in teaching and learning as well as clinical practice (Baldwin et al., 2014). Clinical nurse educators must be cognizant of being watched at all times. Care must be taken to role-model the ideal and not to settle for mediocrity.

## ■ DEMONSTRATING INCLUSIVE EXCELLENCE

*Inclusive excellence* is a term originated by the Association of American Colleges & Universities (AAC&U) and refers to using diversity to promote academic excellence. Since the Institute of Medicine (IOM; as cited in Bleich, MacWilliams, & Schmidt, 2015) declared the need for increasingly diverse healthcare providers, nursing programs have been challenged to meet this demand by increasing the diversity of faculty and students. Although many programs have made changes in an effort to increase the admission and enrollment of a more diverse nursing student body, many of these students are unable to complete the program of study. There likewise is an insufficient number of diverse faculty (Bleich et al., 2015). This makes it incumbent on all clinical nursing faculty to work to create a learning environment that is inclusive and welcoming of diversity.

| 3.2   Evidence-Based Clinical Teaching Practice |
| --- |
| In a study by Tiffany and Hoglund (2016), nurse educator students enrolled in an Inclusivity in Nursing Education course were assigned an avatar in Second Life representing a marginalized person. Results found that because of this exposure, students were better able to understand those who are different. As summed up by one participant, "having the understanding that we all carry certain forms of bias and 'isms' that we need to be aware of is a basis for creating more inclusive nursing education environments" (p. 121). |

Bleich et al. (2015) define *inclusive culture* as "one that brings diverse perspectives into decision-making structures at all levels, allows for and celebrates differences as enriching, and reduces and/or eliminates barriers to full engagement of all" (p. 90). The clinical nurse educator can use different strategies to develop an inclusive culture. It is important that the educator evaluate the CLE to ensure there are opportunities for working with diverse populations. Promoting student-centered learning provides all students with a voice and a say in their learning needs. Creating a learning environment of mutual trust and respect empowers all individuals. The clinical nurse educator may also identify mentors who can serve as positive role models for diverse students. It is especially important to identify and utilize resources and available support when students appear isolated. Although a diverse mentor may be the ideal, a clinical nurse educator who is sensitive to the needs of diverse students and works for inclusiveness can be an effective role model (Bleich et al., 2015).

*Diversity* is often thought to refer to racial or ethnic diversity, but it can also include gender, sexual orientation, gender identity, national origin, religious beliefs, socioeconomic status, and more. The American Association of Colleges of Nursing (as cited in Breslin, Nuri-Robins, Ash, & Kirschling, 2018) defines *inclusion* as a culture in which those who are not part of the dominant culture flourish. It is not merely tolerating those who are different but celebrating the differences they bring to the group. The clinical nurse educator must broaden her or his understanding of diversity to include anyone who is not viewed as mainstream. For the educator to be inclusive, it is important to begin with a self-reflection on personal biases (Breslin et al., 2018). Identifying one's own biases is the first step in moving forward to a more inclusive culture for learners in the CLE.

*Incivility* and *workplace violence* are terms heard all too often in the healthcare setting. The phrase "eating our young" is well known among nurses. *Horizontal violence*, which is lateral aggression or hostile behavior among colleagues, is also well documented in the literature. An example of this is hostile behavior between academic nurses and clinical nurses or between academic faculty and clinical nurse educators. The American Nurses Association (as cited in Schmidt, MacWilliams, & Neal-Boylan, 2016) has found poor health outcomes for patients and nurses to be related to incivility and hostile behaviors in the workplace. It is important for the clinical nurse educator to ensure that students are provided an environment conducive to learning. In settings where incivility and hostile behaviors are common, the educator may need to communicate with the course faculty to identify another more amenable site. When a clinical nurse educator witnesses incivility directed toward students, the issue needs to be addressed directly with the person and secondarily with the nurse manager, if needed. In order to develop an inclusive learning environment for students, the clinical nurse educator needs to be supportive and aware of behaviors that are exclusionary.

---

**3.2   Clinical Nurse Educator Teaching Tip**

Incivility in the workplace is unfortunately not uncommon. Nursing students are particularly vulnerable because they often believe themselves to be powerless. When faced with incivility, many will never address it nor report it, but it can leave a lasting impression. The clinical nurse educator must be aware of the environment and on the lookout for incivility directed toward students. Creating a trusting relationship can empower students to report instances of incivility to the clinical nurse educator. Although instances of incivility may occur in the future, the clinical nurse educator is in a position to address it and to work with students on how to deal with similar issues.

---

## ▪ SUMMARY

As the demand for nurses continues to increase, the need for clinical nurse educators will also continue to climb. The challenge for nursing programs is in finding experienced clinical nurse educators to fill the role. More and more educators are being hired with limited knowledge of nursing education. The challenge is for these novice clinical nurse educators to quickly develop into the role to meet the challenges inherent in functioning as an educator and a practice nurse. Through certification, clinical nurse educators can demonstrate their knowledge and competence of the clinical nurse educator role.

---

**3.1   Case Study**

The prelicensure BSN faculty at a small liberal arts university in the southeastern United States were reviewing how clinical skills were tracked. For years, a paper competency checklist was used for documenting the completion of skills. Faculty expressed concerns that the students were losing the forms and/or forgetting to bring the document to clinical. In keeping with the department's intent to move records to an electronic format, it was suggested that an electronic competency checklist be created. Using funding from a small internal technology grant, a technical expert was hired to develop the document so that students could email a list of the skills they completed to their clinical nurse educator, who in turn could sign-off on skills. Both students and the clinical nurse educators can access this system via smartphone or computer. The new electronic competency checklist was trialed with the new class of students studying nursing fundamentals. During this first semester, both electronic and paper checklists were maintained. The fundamentals' clinical nurse educators and students were oriented by the technical expert on the use of the electronic checklist. As this first group of students moves through the curriculum, additional clinical nurse educators are oriented to the new electronic document. Following each semester of use, the process is reviewed and improvements made.

---

*(continued)*

---

**3.1  Case Study (*continued*)**

Questions for Reflection:

- Identify factors that would enable the clinical nurse educator to accurately utilize this new technology.
- Analyze potential detriments to the clinical nurse educator comfortably using this new technology.
- Evaluate different strategies the clinical nurse educator can use when dealing with students resistant to implementation of this new technology.
- Develop a plan that the clinical nurse educator can use in working with professional nursing staff who have a negative view of mobile devices in the CLE.

CLE, clinical learning environment.

---

## ▓ REVIEW QUESTIONS

1. An elderly patient admitted with a urinary tract infection is demonstrating deterioration in his status. When speaking to the patient's student nurse, the clinical nurse educator discusses her own assessment of the situation and rationales for further interventions. This is an example of:

   A. Psychomotor apprenticeship

   B. Cognitive apprenticeship

   C. Socratic questioning

   D. Autocratic instruction

2. A new clinical nurse educator is relating to his mentor how he coached a student today. What statement would indicate that the educator needs further information on coaching?

   A. "My student observed me providing instructions on insulin administration today."

   B. "Instead of directly answering questions, I had my student look up the answer."

   C. "I required my student to explain the rationale for each of her interventions."

   D. "I observed my student perform her assessment and then I provided feedback."

3. An experienced clinical nurse educator is working to better motivate her students. How can the educator influence the student who is extrinsically motivated?

   A. Assign a letter grade as part of the feedback on concept maps.

   B. Praise the student after completing new skills.

   C. List areas for improvement following a procedure.

   D. Assign a challenging dressing change that the student has performed previously.

4. A clinical nurse educator expresses to her mentor an interest in using debriefing in postconferences. Which statement by the clinical nurse educator indicates an accurate understanding of the debriefing process?

A. "Debriefing is a simple process that can be done in a few minutes."

B. "Debriefing focuses on highlighting all that was done incorrectly by the student."

C. "During the debriefing, I will be reflecting on what could have been done differently."

D. "In order to be effective with my debriefing, I will first seek training opportunities."

5. Students have been assigned to keep a reflective journal of their clinical experiences. What statement by the novice clinical nurse educator would indicate that further instruction is needed relative to the reflective journals?

A. "It is important that a trusting relationship be developed so students will feel safe in documenting their feelings."

B. "Changes in attitudes should be noted early in the reflective journaling process."

C. "When reading their journals, it is important to remain nonjudgmental."

D. "Students need instruction on the purpose and benefits of reflective journaling."

6. A clinical nurse educator is planning an assignment that will promote leadership skills. Which assignment would be most effective?

A. Instruct the student to delegate non-nursing tasks to the unlicensed assistive personnel.

B. Assign the student to observe the charge nurse for the day.

C. Assign the student to perform complete care for the patient.

D. Inform the student he will be administering medications to his patient today.

7. A nurse manager is overheard talking about students being on their phones in the clinical learning environment (CLE). What action by the clinical nurse educator would be least helpful in this situation?

A. Check the agency policy to ensure students are not in violation.

B. Meet privately with the nurse manager to address her concerns.

C. Inform the nurse manager that this is the future of technology in practice.

D. Monitor the students' phone usage to ensure they are not on social media.

8. A clinical nurse educator is talking to a colleague about the use of mobile devices in the clinical learning environment (CLE). Which statement provides the best argument for its use?

A. "Students have access to a multitude of references allowing them to search for the current, best evidence."

B. "Students and faculty can continue to access email and remain connected to their courses and instructors."

    C. "The professional nursing staff are constantly using their phones, so there is no reason the students shouldn't as well."

    D. "Students are more engaged when they are using their phones and working as a team."

9. A clinical nurse educator is trying to ensure inclusive excellence in the clinical learning environment (CLE). What action would be most effective in achieving this?

    A. Ask all students in postconference to discuss their ethnic background.

    B. Require all students to speak up during postconference activities.

    C. Provide students with the opportunity to speak openly and freely in postconference.

    D. Invite a minority nurse to speak to the students in postconference.

10. A student is observed sitting at the nurse's station using a smartphone while call lights are ringing. What would be the best response for the clinical nurse educator?

    A. Take the student's phone for the remainder of the clinical day.

    B. Privately meet with the student to discuss appropriate use of the smartphone.

    C. Inform the student that she will be receiving a clinical warning.

    D. Prohibit smartphone use in the clinical learning environment (CLE) for the rest of the semester.

## ▨ REFERENCES

AL Sabei, S. D., & Lasater, K. (2016). Simulation debriefing for clinical judgment development: A concept analysis. *Nurse Education Today, 45*, 42–47. doi:10.1016/j.nedt.2016.06.008

Baldwin, A., Mills, J., Birks, M., & Budden, L. (2014). Role modeling in undergraduate nursing education: An integrative literature review. *Nurse Education Today, 34*, e18–e26. doi:10.1016/j.nedt.2013.12.007

Battle, L. H., & Tyson, T. (2018). Academic strategies that facilitate learning in millennial nursing students. *I-manager's Journal on Nursing, 8*(1), 1–10. doi:10.1016/j.profnurs.2016.08.004

Bleich, M. R., MacWilliams, B. R., & Schmidt, B. J. (2015). Advancing diversity through inclusive excellence in nursing education. *Journal of Professional Nursing, 31*(2), 89–94. doi:10.1016/j.profnurs.2014.09.003

Breslin, E. T., Nuri-Robins, K., Ash, J., & Kirschling, J. M. (2018). The changing face of academic nursing: Nurturing diversity, inclusivity, and equity. *Journal of Professional Nursing, 34*, 103–109. doi:10.1016/j.profnurs.2017.12.014

Cho, S., & Lee, E. (2016). Distraction by smartphone use during clinical practice and opinions about smartphone restriction policies: A cross-sectional descriptive study of nursing students. *Nurse Education Today, 40*, 128–133. doi:10.1016/j.nedt.2016.02.021

Demeh, W., & Rosengren, K. (2015). The visualisation of clinical leadership in the content of nursing education: A qualitative study of nursing students' experiences. *Nurse Education Today, 35*(7), 888–893.

Dewitty, V. P., Huerta, C. G., & Downing, C. A. (2016). New careers in nursing: Optimizing diversity and student success for the future of nursing. *Journal of Professional Nursing, 32*(5S), S4–S13. doi:10.1016/j.profnurs.2016.03.011

Dufrene, C., & Young, A. (2014). Successful debriefing—Best methods to achieve positive learning outcomes: A literature review. *Nurse Education Today, 34*, 372–376. doi:10.1016/j.nedt.2013.06.026

Felstead, I. S., & Springett, K. (2016). An exploration of role model influence on adult nursing students' professional development: A phenomenological research study. *Nurse Education Today, 37*, 66–70. doi:10.1016/j.nedt.2015.11.014

Fiedler, R., Giddens, J., & North, S. (2014). Faculty experience of a technological innovation in nursing education. *Nursing Education Perspectives, 35*(6), 387–391. doi:10.5480/13-1188

Forneris, S. G., Neal, D. O., Tiffany, J., Kuehn, M. B., Meyer, H. M., Blazovich, L. M., . . . Smerillo, M. (2015). Enhancing clinical reasoning through simulation debriefing: A multisite study. *Nursing Education Perspectives, 36*(5), 304–310. doi:10.5480/15-1672

Gantt, L. T., Overton, S. H., Avery, J., Swanson, M., & Elhammoumi, C. V. (2018). Comparison of debriefing methods and learning outcomes in human patient simulation. *Clinical Simulation in Nursing, 17,* 7–13. doi:10.1016/j.ecns.2017.11.012

Gunay, U., & Kilinc, G. (2018). The transfer of theoretical knowledge to clinical practice by nursing students and the difficulties they experience: A qualitative study. *Nurse Education Today, 65,* 81–86. doi:10.1016/j.nedt.2018.02.031

Kang, K., & Yu, M. (2018). Comparison of student self-debriefing versus instructor debriefing in nursing simulation: A quasi-experimental study. *Nurse Education Today, 65,* 67–73. doi:10.1016/j.nedt.2018.02.030

Lavoie, P., Pepin, J., & Cossette, S. (2017). Contribution of a reflective debriefing to nursing students' clinical judgment in patient deterioration simulations: A mixed-methods study. *Nurse Education Today, 50,* 51–56. doi:10.1016/j.nedt.2016.12.002

Lyons, K., McLaughlin, J. E., Khanova, J., & Roth, M. T. (2017). Cognitive apprenticeship in health sciences education: A qualitative review. *Advances in Health Sciences Education, 22,* 723–739. doi:10.1007/s10459-016-9707-4

Mackay, B. J., Anderson, J., & Harding, T. (2017). Mobile technology in clinical teaching. *Nurse Education in Practice, 22,* 1–6. doi:10.1016/j.nepr.2016.11.001

Mahlanze, H. T., & Sibiya, M. N. (2017). Perceptions of student nurses on the writing of reflective journals as a means for personal, professional and clinical learning development. *Health SA Gesondheid – Journal of Interdisciplinary Health Sciences, 22,* 79–86. doi:10.1016/j.hsag.2016.05.005

McNally, G., Frey, R., & Crossan, M. (2017). Nurse manager and student nurse perceptions of the use of personal smartphones or tablets and the adjunct applications, as an educational tool in clinical settings. *Nurse Education in Practice, 23,* 1–7. doi:10.1016/j.nepr.2016.12.004

Patterson, E. E. B., Boyd, L., & Mnatzaganian, G. (2017). The impact of undergraduate clinical teaching models on the perceptions of work-readiness among new graduate nurses: A cross sectional study. *Nurse Education Today, 55,* 101–106. doi:10.1016/j.nedt.2017.05.010

Raymond, C., Profetto-McGrath, J., Myrick, F., & Strean, W. B. (2018). Balancing the seen and unseen: Nurse educator as role model for critical thinking. *Nurse Education in Practice, 31,* 41–47. doi:10.1016/j.nepr.2018.04.010

Risling, T. (2017). Educating the nurses of 2025: Technology trends of the next decade. *Nurse Education in Practice, 22,* 89–92. doi:10.1016/j.nepr.2016.12.007

Roberts, D., & Williams, A. (2017). The potential of mobile technology (#MoTech) to close the theory practice gap. *Nurse Education Today, 53,* 26–28. doi:10.1016/j.nedt.2017.03.003

Schmidt, B. J., MacWilliams, B. R., & Neal-Boylan, L. (2016). Becoming inclusive: A code of conduct for inclusion and diversity. *Journal of Professional Nursing, 33*(2), 102–107. doi:10.1016/j.profnurs.2016.08.014

Tiffany, J. M., & Hoglund, B. A. (2016). Using virtual simulation to teach inclusivity: A case study. *Clinical Simulation in Nursing, 12,* 115–122. doi:10.1016/j.ecns.2015.11.003

Walker, R., Cooke, M., Henderson, A., & Creedy, D. K. (2011). Characteristics of leadership that influence clinical learning: A narrative review. *Nurse Education Today, 31,* 743–756. doi:10.1016/j.nedt.2010.12.018

# 4

# Functioning Within the Education and Healthcare Environments: Operationalize the Curriculum

*LINDA WILSON*

*I think the big thing is don't be afraid to fail. It's a part of building character and growing.*
—Nick Foles

## ■ LEARNING OUTCOMES

At the end of this chapter, the learner will be able to

- Discuss the importance of congruence between the clinical site and the curriculum.
- Describe the development of relevant clinical assignments and activities.
- Review preparation of the student for clinical experiences.
- Review interprofessional collaboration.
- Discuss strategies for developing problem-solving skills.

## ■ INTRODUCTION

The curriculum can be operationalized in a variety of places where the student can interact with patients, families, and communities. The clinical learning environment (CLE) can influence learning outcomes and provide opportunities for integrating knowledge, promoting clinical judgment, and professional identity (Billings & Halstead, 2016). Practice environments must be supportive so that learners can develop necessary skills to ensure competency (O'Mara, McDonald, Gillespie, Brown,

& Miles, 2014). Oermann, Shellenbarger, and Gaberson (2018) identified five main components of clinical teaching:

1. Identify learning outcomes.
2. Assess learning needs.
3. Plan learning activities.
4. Guide learners.
5. Evaluate outcomes.

## ▓ ASSESS CONGRUENCE OF THE CLINICAL AGENCY TO CURRICULUM

The curriculum is designed to promote continuous knowledge building. Clinical experiences must be planned so that they are congruent with the curriculum and learner outcomes. Patient experiences should be planned so that they enhance or supplement what was learned in theory each week. As the learner progresses the faculty needs to interpret the curriculum and identify appropriate clinical experiences (Billings & Halstead, 2016).

### Course Goals

The clinical nurse educator must be familiar with the course goals so that appropriate clinical experiences can be planned. Implementing clinical activities can be challenging due to many factors, including

1. High demand for clinical sites
2. Competition to confirm clinical sites
3. Increased number of nursing and other health professions learners, which can overwhelm a clinical environment (Oermann et al., 2018).

### Learner Needs

Clinical experiences provide learners the opportunity to practice all aspects of nursing. The academic clinical nurse educator must identify each learner's needs and provide optimal clinical experiences to meet those needs. To achieve the best results, the faculty must have knowledge of each learner and her or his specific needs. The initial assessment by the academic clinical faculty is to examine the learner's prerequisite knowledge and skills for the clinical experience (Oermann et al., 2018). If a lack of knowledge is identified, the learner can be recommended for remediation. The academic clinical faculty must also consider the individual characteristics of each learner, including learning styles, cultural background, age, life experiences, generational differences, and many others (Oermann et al., 2018). The clinical learning activities should build on the learner's knowledge and experience and consider other learner attributes (Oermann et al., 2018).

## Plan Meaningful and Relevant Clinical Learning Assignments

When planning clinical learning activities, the priorities include the following:

1. Competencies to be learned
2. Learner outcomes
3. Individual learner needs
4. Effectiveness of learning activities
5. The clinical environment
6. Teacher availability to guide learners (Oermann et al., 2018); clinical experiences need to be consistent with the course and expected learner outcomes; clinical assignments should be planned so that they enhance what was learned in the theory portion of the class each week; patient assignments should increase in number and complexity as the course proceeds

## Simulation

Simulation is an excellent method to use to provide clinical experiences that a learner might not have the opportunity to see while in the clinical setting. There are numerous simulation techniques that can be used for these learning experiences, including

1. Human patient simulator simulation
2. Standardized patient simulation
3. Hybrid simulation
4. Task-trainer simulation
5. Virtual-reality simulation

Simulation provides the opportunity to learn in a safe environment that is very realistic to actual clinical experiences. Simulation can also provide experiences in interprofessional collaboration and therapeutic communication. Complex simulation scenarios can also provide learner opportunities for critical thinking/clinical judgment.

| 4.1  Clinical Nurse Educator Teaching Tip |
|---|
| Standardized patient simulation includes the use of patient actors. The use of patient actors can provide the most realistic simulation because the actors can portray emotions, complex communication, and even challenging ethical dilemmas. |

## Evidence-Based Practice Activities

Evidence-based practice (EBP) activities can provide the learner with the opportunity to identify a clinical problem or clinical challenge and to use current evidence to solve that challenge. There are numerous EBP models that can be used for this activity, including the following:

1. Johns Hopkins Model (Newhouse, Dearholt, Poe, Pugh, & White, 2007)
2. Iowa Model (Iowa Model Collaborative, 2017)
3. JBI Model (Jordan, Lockwood, Aromataris, & Munn, 2016)
4. Star Model (Stevens, 2012)

Clinical learners can work individually or in groups on this learning activity.

---

**4.2  Clinical Nurse Educator Teaching Tip**

EBP models can initially be confusing to learners. The Johns Hopkins Model (Newhouse et al., 2007) is an excellent EBP model to start with because it is presented in a clear, easy-to-understand format.

EBP, evidence-based practice.

---

**4.1  Evidence-Based Clinical Teaching Practice**

The Iowa Model Collaborative (2017) examined the use of the original model and synthesized information and recommendations before revising the Iowa Model of EBP. Use of the model was requested by 431 people between 2001 and 2013. Of those who requested access, 83% ($n = 379$) used the model and identified challenges with its use. With this feedback, the Iowa Model was revised and then evaluated by participants ($n = 299$). The new model was then validated as an EBP tool across multiple settings.

EBP, evidence-based practice.

---

## ▦ PREPARE LEARNERS

### Clinical Orientation

Prior to or on the first clinical day, a comprehensive clinical site orientation should be provided to the learners. The orientation should include the following:

1. Orientation to the specific clinical unit
2. Orientation to the various clinical departments
3. Orientation to emergency codes and procedures
4. Review of policies, procedures, and the student handbook
5. Review of expectations for the clinical

6. Review of expected learner outcomes

7. Clinical documentation

8. Procedures for medication administration

9. Process for completion of bedside procedures

10. What to do if an error occurs

## ▨ ELECTRONIC MEDICAL RECORD

If a clinical facility has an electronic medical record (EMR), and the clinical learners are permitted to document in the EMR, a comprehensive training on the use of the EMR should be provided for the faculty and the learners. Several companies have developed academic EMRs that can be incorporated into the curriculum. Several barriers exist with implementing an academic EMR, including the following:

1. Cost of the technology

2. Training time for faculty and learners

3. The academic EMRs do not depict all EMRs used in healthcare settings today (Oermann et al., 2018)

## ▨ STRUCTURE LEARNER EXPERIENCES

### Clinical Assignments

Patient assignments should be planned so that they augment what is learned in the theory portion of the course each week. Initially, each clinical student should be assigned one patient so that the academic clinical educator can assess the communication skills, physical exam skills, and problem-solving skills of each student. Once this is assessed, the academic clinical educator can assign appropriate clinical patient experiences for each student. As the course progresses, the number of patients assigned to each student should increase as should the patients' case complexity.

### Preceptor in Specialty Environments

Assigning the students a preceptor in a specialty unit is another excellent learning experience. This opportunity, even if for observation only, can provide the learner with exposure to other nursing roles and specialties in nursing. Some specialty preceptors to consider are the following:

1. Post anesthesia care unit

2. Operating room

3. Preadmission testing area

4. Interventional radiology

5. Endoscopy

6. Emergency department

7. Critical care units

8. Trauma unit (as well as many other areas)

## ▦ DEDICATED EDUCATIONAL UNITS

Some clinical facilities have developed dedicated educational units (DEU) that promote clinical education and experiences. In the DEU, the staff nurses are the learners' clinical instructors (Wittmann-Price, Godshall, & Wilson, 2017). The nurses who work in DEUs are supportive of the educational process and are eager to work with students. The DEU provides a very positive learning environment for students.

---

**4.2   Evidence-Based Clinical Teaching Practice**

Carey, Kent, and Latour (2018) conducted a qualitative systematic review to examine peer-assisted learning in clinical practice for undergraduate nursing students. Eight studies were identified and 37 findings were extracted and then these findings were further analyzed to produce three synthesized findings. "These three findings include: 1) challenges of clinical practices are mitigated by peer support; 2) peers are role models for enhancing clinical knowledge; and 3) support and feedback develop competence and confidence and reduce stress and anxiety" (p. 1190).

---

### Help Learners Develop Interprofessional Collaboration

Interprofessional clinical experiences can teach learners how to work collaboratively with other healthcare disciplines. There are many opportunities in the clinical environment for the student to observe interprofessional collaboration. Interprofessional collaboration can be observed in all clinical units, but some particularly excellent examples include: (a) operating room, (b) rapid response team, (c) code team, and (d) trauma team. The outcome of interprofessional clinical experiences should be the development of teamwork competencies (Billings & Halstead, 2016).

### TeamSTEPPS

TeamSTEPPS is a teamwork system developed by the Agency for Healthcare Research and Quality (AHRQ, 2018). TeamSTEPPS training was designed to improve quality and safety in healthcare by focusing on the core teamwork skills of communication, leadership, situation monitoring, and mutual support (AHRQ, 2018). TeamSTEPPS can be incorporated in clinical experiences and simulation experiences.

### Develop Problem-Solving Capability

*Critical thinking/clinical judgment* can be fostered through a variety of learning activities such as case studies, problem-solving, and reflective thinking. Case studies provide the opportunity for the learner to examine a clinical situation and to identify appropriate assessment and interventions. Problem-solving techniques encourage the learner to identify a problem, gather information, identify interventions, and choose the best action to take (Oermann et al., 2018).

*Reflective thinking* allows the learner to consider multiple options when approaching the patient situation, identify which approach is best based on evidence, clarify questions to ask to obtain additional information, and then determine the best approach to use in the situation (Oermann et al., 2018). Tanner (2006) describes the clinical judgment process in four parts:

1. Grasp the situation.
2. Interpret the situation.
3. Decide on appropriate actions.
4. Reflect on the patient's response.

### Provide Input to the Nursing Program

CLEs should have representation on the advisory boards for nursing schools because they can provide insight on current clinical practice, challenges, expectations, and innovations. Nursing programs should survey graduates to solicit their feedback on the nursing program as well as their success in job acquisition. Nursing schools should survey employers for feedback on how new graduates are working out in the clinical setting. Academic clinical instructors should provide feedback to the school of nursing and to the clinical site on the clinical experiences, supportiveness of staff, and the overall environment.

### ▩ SUMMARY

The role of the academic clinical nurse educator is a very important one for the nursing program, the learners, and the clinical site. It is imperative for the academic clinical nurse educator to be knowledgeable about the curriculum and learner outcomes in order to facilitate a successful clinical experience for the learners.

---

**4.1 Case Study**

The academic clinical nurse educator has preplanned the clinical assignments for the learners on the unit today. Upon arrival to the unit on the morning of the clinical, the academic

*(continued)*

---

**4.1  Case Study (*continued*)**

nurse educator learns that several of the patients needed for the planned patient assignments have been transferred or discharged. What should the academic clinical nurse educator do?

The academic clinical nurse educator has several options: (a) assign several students to work together on a complex patient, (b) identify an observational experience for some students in a specialty unit such as the ED or post anesthesia care unit, or (c) identify a shadowing experience with a specialty nursing role such as a diabetes educator.

**Questions for Reflection:**

How would each assignment meet the student learning outcomes?

How does the clinical nurse educator monitor the students' activities?

How does the clinical nurse educator ensure that assignments do not use discharged patients, if possible?

---

## ▩ REVIEW QUESTIONS

1. The clinical nurse educator plans to use an educational activity to have the students demonstrate postoperative assessment techniques. Which activity will be the most effective?

   A. Case study report of a postoperative patient

   B. Simulation activity using the human patient simulator

   C. Literature review of therapeutic communication

   D. Computer simulation of a postoperative patient

2. The clinical educator wants to evaluate the therapeutic communication of the learners. Which activity will be the most effective?

   A. Case study report of a postoperative patient

   B. Simulation activity using a standardized patient

   C. Literature review of postoperative care

   D. Computer simulation of a postoperative patient

3. Which of the following can be implemented during orientation to a new clinical learning environment to best reach the goal of familiarizing students with the type of patients on the unit?

   A. Treasure hunt

   B. Electronic medical records (EMR) training

   C. Review of medical records and documentation

   D. Introducing students to patients

4. Which one of the following techniques includes clarifying questions to help determine the best approach?

   A. Case studies

   B. Problem-based learning

   C. Reflective learning

   D. Socratic questioning

5. The best explanation a clinical nurse educator can provide students about TeamSTEPPS is:

  A. An analysis process used by individuals in the clinical setting

  B. A research process used for evidence-based practice

  C. A teamwork system developed by the Agency for Healthcare Research and Quality

  D. An evidence-based practice process developed by the Agency for Healthcare Research and Quality

6. The clinical nurse educator understands that a student who is reluctant to call the primary care provider about a needed medication change should be:

  A. Instructed to leave the unit because the student is unprepared

  B. Remediated about TeamSTEPPS

  C. Provided with a clinical warning and a learning plan

  D. Taken to the simulation laboratory for practice

7. A novice nurse educator states that use of electronic medical records (EMRs) should be taught after students learn how to document longhand because that is the way she learned and it was useful. The best recommendation to the novice nurse educator is to:

  A. Tell her that longhand documentation is outdated.

  B. Inform her that the school uses only EMR documentation.

  C. She should explain both methods to students.

  D. She should participate in the skills laboratory when students are being orientated to documentation.

8. A novice nurse educator assigns students to specialty units for multiple days during the medical course. The course instructor should review what with the novice educator?

  A. The student learning outcomes for the course

  B. The skills the students should know

  C. The old clinical schedules

  D. Her philosophy of hands-on education

9. Dedicated education units (DEUs) have improved learner outcomes by:

  A. Having learners do evidence-based projects

  B. Reassigning the same patients to students

  C. Having a consistent, educated preceptor

  D. Having independence in the student role

10. Congruency in clinical placement to the adult–gerontology healthy aging course would be:

  A. An acute care facility

  B. A long-term care facility

  C. Outpatient facility

  D. Adult day care

▨ **REFERENCES**

Agency for Healthcare Research and Quality. (2018). About TeamSTEPPS. Retrieved from https://www.ahrq.gov/teamstepps/about-teamstepps/index.html

Billings, D. M., & Halstead, J. A. (2016). *Teaching in nursing: A guide for faculty* (5th ed.). St. Louis, MO: Elsevier.

Carey, M. C., Kent, B., & Latour, J. M. (2018). Experiences of undergraduate nursing students in peer assisted learning in clinical practice: A qualitative systematic review. *JBI Database of Systematic Reviews and Implementation Reports, 16*(5), 1190–1219.

Iowa Model Collaborative. (2017). Iowa model of evidence-based practice: Revisions and validation. *Worldviews on Evidence-Based Nursing, 14*(3), 175–182.

Jordan, Z., Lockwood, C., Aromataris, E., & Munn, Z. (2016). *The updated Joanna Briggs Institute model for evidence-based healthcare.* Retrieved from https://www.researchgate.net/publication/327914760_The_updated_Joanna_Briggs_Institute_Model_of_Evidence-Based_Healthcare:

Newhouse, R. P., Dearholt, S. L., Poe, S. S., Pugh, L. C., & White, K. (2007). *Johns Hopkins nursing evidence-based practice model and guidelines.* Indianapolis, IN: Sigma Theta Tau International.

Oermann, M. H., Shellenbarger, T., & Gaberson, K. B. (2018). *Clinical teaching strategies in nursing* (5th ed.). New York, NY: Springer Publishing Company.

O'Mara, L., McDonald, J., Gillespie, M., Brown, H., & Miles, L. (2014). Challenging clinical learning environments: Experiences of undergraduate nursing students. *Nurse Education in Practice, 14*(2), 208–213.

Stevens, K. R. (2012). *Star model of EBP: Knowledge transformation.* Academic Center for Evidence-based Practice. San Antonio, TX: The University of Texas Health Science Center.

Tanner, C. A. (2006). Thinking like a nurse: A research-based model of clinical judgement in nursing. *Journal of Nursing Education, 45,* 204–211.

Wittmann-Price, R., Godshall, M., & Wilson, L. (2017). *Certified nurse educator (CNE) review manual* (3rd ed.). New York, NY: Springer Publishing Company.

# 5

# Functioning Within the Education and Healthcare Environments: Abide by Legal Requirements, Ethical Guidelines, Agency Policies, and Guiding Framework

MARY ELLEN SMITH GLASGOW

*The most important human endeavor is the striving for morality in our actions.*
*Our inner balance and even our very existence depend on it. Only*
*morality in our actions can give beauty and dignity to life.*
—Albe Eins

## ■ LEARNING OUTCOMES

At the end of this chapter, the learner will be able to

- Discuss the legal and ethical issues pertaining to the role of a nursing faculty member in the clinical environment.
- Apply a "just culture" framework to clinical nursing education.
- Discuss internal and external factors impacting clinical nursing education.
- Analyze a case study with the legal, ethical, and agency policies and "just culture" framework in mind.

## ■ INTRODUCTION

Clinical nursing education is a critical component of basic and advanced practice nursing education. Clinical teaching begins with clinical nurse educators who have a full understanding of the clinical objectives for the clinical learning experience (CLE) and a clear understanding of the benchmarks, daily objectives, or progressive objectives that gauge students' progress toward these objectives (Gardner & Suplee, 2010). Evaluation involves the clinical nurse educator's assessment of the student's performance, which may involve some subjectivity, as one person is observing another (Brown, Neudorf, Poitras, & Rodger, 2007).

A clinical evaluation plan includes both formative and summative evaluations, a daily plan with clear daily performance objectives that are clearly related to the overall clinical objectives for the rotation and unbiased, iterative, daily feedback to each student about clinical performance, including opportunities for improvement. Clinical nurse educators should keep documentation of each student's progress via weekly summaries and incident-specific anecdotal notes (Gardner & Suplee, 2010). There are numerous internal and external forces impacting the practice of the clinical nurse educator: clinical agency policies and procedures, academic policies, compliance with regulations and standards of practice, institutional mission/values, and ethical professional practice. Novice clinical nurse educators face a particularly steep learning curve and new challenges as they enter the academy, and even more so if their graduate education did not have specific coursework on the teaching role. Efforts need to be made to mitigate the knowledge deficits related to clinical nursing education pedagogy and evaluation.

## ▪ APPLYING ETHICAL AND LEGAL PRINCIPLES WHEN PLANNING CLINICAL LEGAL EXPERIENCES

Clinical nurse educators need to do a fair amount of preparation before the first clinical day. The clinical nurse educator needs to familiarize himself or herself with the course syllabus, clinical evaluation tool, academic policies, clinical agency policies and practices, practice environment, and appropriate clinical nursing education pedagogies (clinical assignment making, preconference, postconference, simulation, debriefing, reflection, and evaluation). Clinical nurse orientation should acknowledge the clinical nurse educator's expectations and needs including (a) academic skills—development of instructional skills, integration into the culture of higher education, development of skills for locating information and managing the clinical academic workload and (b) supports—creation of an ongoing development plan to support the clinical nurse educators who is somewhat isolated from the academic institution (Santisteban & Egues, 2014; Suplee & Gardner, 2009).

## ▪ ASSESSING LEARNERS' ABILITIES

The clinical nurse educator assesses student learners' abilities and needs prior to CLEs and informs the students of applicable clinical policies and standards. Clinical nurse educators should assess the student in preparation for the clinical experience. Preclinical conference is a practical way to assess student preparedness for the clinical experience. If it is determined that the student is unprepared, the student should not be assigned to a patient for care activities (Strader, 1985). Preclinical

and postclinical conferences afford students and clinical nurse educators an opportunity to address student questions and discuss challenging patient care assignments in a safe, learning environment (Patton &
Lewallen, 2015).

## SUPPORTING THE MISSION

Clinical nurse educators also need to be cognizant and in alignment
with the mission and values of the academic institution and clinical
agency and be proficient with the ever-changing healthcare technology
landscape.

---

**5.1 Evidence-Based Clinical Teaching Practice**

Andrew, Halcomb, Jackson, Peters, and Salamonson (2010) found that clinical nurse educators who teach using current practice examples to teach students the "real" world of practice
are bridging the current reality practice gap. By sharing their own clinical practice stories,
reflecting upon their own experiences, and providing examples stemming from their own
clinical experiences, clinical nurse educators are helping students integrate knowledge into
their own clinical experiences.

---

## INFORMING OTHERS OF POLICIES

Clinical nurse educators should be familiar with the Quality and
Safety Education for Nurses (QSEN) competencies (additional information about QSEN is located in Chapter 6, Facilitate Learning
in the Healthcare Environment, and Chapter 8, Apply Clinical
Expertise in the Healthcare Environment). Clinical nurse educators must be able to differentiate between errors and near misses,
human error and system failure, and at-risk and reckless behaviors
(Barnsteiner & Disch, 2017a). In order to have effective clinical learning,
students need to feel safe and supported, and they also must clearly
understand the ground rules.

Recently, Barnsteiner and Disch (2017a) applied a *just culture* framework to clinical nursing education. A *just culture* can be described as a
fair, balanced approach to event reporting, learning from mistakes, and
holding persons and the organization accountable. This just culture is
the context wherein students learn and improve by openly identifying
and examining their weaknesses and feeling supported in doing so—
this is described as a just clinical learning environment (Marx, 2001).

The notion of fairness is integral to a fair and Just Culture. It is
understood that mistakes will occur, and that having a shared
accountability model in place promotes both individual- and
system-level learning from those mistakes. Individuals know

they will be held accountable for their actions, but will not be blamed for system faults that lie beyond their control. Errors and inappropriate clinical behavior can be categorized as human error, at-risk behaviors, and reckless behaviors. (Barnsteiner & Disch, 2017b, p. 42)

In this atmosphere of trust, students are encouraged, even rewarded, for providing essential safety information—however, there is a clear line between acceptable and unacceptable behavior (Reason, 1997; Additional information about just culture is provided in Chapter 8, Apply Clinical Expertise in the Healthcare Environment).

*Human error* is described as inadvertently doing other than what should have been done—a slip, lapse, or mistake. For example, if a student misreads a medication label due to a distraction resulting in a near-miss medication error, the clinical nurse educator addresses and acknowledges this error. *At-risk behavior* is a behavioral choice that increases risk in which risk is not recognized or is mistakenly believed to be justified. For example, a student did not check the patient's identification bracelet before medication administration because he or she did not want to disrupt the patient's sleep. The hospital recently conducted a campaign on promoting patient rest and sleep; thus giving mixed signals to the student. The clinical nurse educator provides remediation. *Reckless behavior* is a behavioral choice to consciously disregard a substantial and unjustifiable risk; for example, if the student enters the clinical environment intoxicated, disciplinary sanctions are applied. Human error (first error) would *generally* require coaching, whereas at-risk behavior would require remediation (Barnsteiner & Disch, 2017b; Boysen, 2013; Dekker, 2008). Reckless behavior for students engaged in a clinical practicum would include the following:

- Being unprepared
- Failing to seek remediation when advised to do so
- Disregarding clinical policies or safe practice
- Failing to raise or report a safety concern
- Speaking or acting disrespectfully toward another person
- Engaging in or tolerating abusive, bullying behaviors
- Looking up or discussing private information about patients outside of specified patient assignment/responsibilities
- Attending clinical while impaired by any substance or condition that compromises one's ability to function safely
- Reporting false positive information to faculty to gain favor (Barnsteiner & Disch, 2017a)

The student engaged in reckless behavior requires due process, which is addressed in the following section. If the reckless behavior is substantiated, the student requires disciplinary action appropriate to the infraction ranging from a warning to dismissal.

## ■ ADHERING TO POLICIES

Because of their subjectivity, students often challenge clinical evaluations. It is crucial that clinical faculty understand the student's right to due process (Whitney, 2009). In very general terms, the "right to due process" equates with fairness. In education, the nursing program or college satisfies this right by stipulating in writing the policies and procedures expected in student performance. Applied to a university's clinical settings, *due process* has been interpreted to mean that a student:

1. Has ample opportunity of notice of misconduct or performance.

2. Is given suggestions for improvement.

3. Is advised of the consequences for failure to improve.

It is to be predicted that there will be disagreement about whether this process was followed, therefore documentation is essential. Standards for theory, clinical objectives, and performance must be provided to students at the start of each semester (Smith Glasgow, Dreher, & Oxholm, 2012).

The fifth and 14th amendments of the U.S. Constitution guarantee citizens "due process of law" and assert to fairness of the government in application of laws to citizens. *Substantive due process* refers to basic fairness, and *procedural due process* is the set of procedural safeguards that are established in protection of individual liberty or property of interest. And, more specifically, most faculty (nor students) do not know that private institutions do not have to follow the protections of due process as these constitutional protections only technically apply to state or federal institutions (e.g., Air Force Academy). Instead, private institutions use internal procedures that closely mimic due process procedures without identifying them as such (Kaplin & Lee, 2013).

## ■ PROMOTING LEARNER COMPLIANCE

In education, the nursing program or college must stipulate in writing—in the form of policies—what the procedural safeguards and guidelines are and how issues of academic misconduct or performance will be treated. Such procedural guidelines should ensure that students are given the opportunities to be heard, review the charges and evidence against them, appear before an impartial decision maker, and appeal the decision (Lindsay, 2005; Roth, 2007).

Due process rights, even in cases involving students, require faculty decisions to be careful and deliberate (Kaplin & Lee, 2013;

Smith, McKoy, & Richardson, 2001). Due process is sustained when faculty have ample documentation and have provided notice to the student with recommendations for improvement and information regarding the student's right to appeal (Suplee, Lachman, & Seibert, 2008). Recording students' activities on each clinical day by keeping meticulous anecdotal notes—accomplishments, performance issues, discipline conferences—is essential (Gardner & Suplee, 2010).

## ▧ DEMONSTRATE ETHICAL BEHAVIOR

Students and faculty reflect the image of the educational institution. A breach of expected conduct, whether covert or overt, reflects poorly on the nursing program and can place the institution in a precarious predicament (Johnson, 2009). Standards for theory, clinical objectives, and performance must be provided to students at the start of each semester. Students must be informed that their student status is analogous to all nurses in maintaining a professional standard of care as delineated in the American Nurses Association's *Code of Ethics* (Johnson, 2009). Students' practice expectations should be addressed in the course syllabus or handbook to include respectful behavior, communication, and clinical preparation, as well as professional responsibilities to faculty, professional nursing staff, ancillary clinical employees, patients, and families (Whitney, 2009). Conduct that is not within acceptable limits should also be addressed in the nursing student handbook, course syllabi, and clinical evaluation tools.

Misconduct can range from emotional outbursts, incivility, and lack of integrity to acts of poor judgment. In the CLE, students may demonstrate misconduct by:

- Being unprepared for clinical assignments
- Disrespecting staff or patients
- Displaying an inability to manage the stressors related to clinical performance (Smith et al., 2001)

Student nurses' misconduct may jeopardize the health and welfare of patients. To ensure safe clinicians, clinical nurse educators have a legal responsibility to convey unsatisfactory grades to students who are not capable of meeting standards of nursing practice; in doing so, clinical nurse educators must also remember to provide due process to students at the same time (Patton & Lewallen, 2015; Smith et al., 2001).

Students must know at the very beginning of their clinical rotations the expected behaviors as well as the consequences if they fail to meet them (Kolanko et al., 2006). Faculty versed in the concept of fairness and just decisions regarding clinical evaluations are acting responsibly on behalf of the public they serve (Smith Glasgow & Dreher, 2007). When misconduct failures or dismissals are enacted, clinical faculty must take several steps to ensure that the student's right to due process is maintained (Johnson, 2009). These steps are listed in Exhibit 5.1.

---

**Exhibit 5.1  Steps to Ensure Due Process**

1. Develop clear policies related to student appeal processes.
2. The student is entitled to written notice of any charges against him or her.
3. The student is provided sufficient opportunity to rebut the charges.
4. The student has a right to select an advisor (if stipulated in the program or college policy).
5. The student has a right to confront his or her accusers.
6. The student has a right to present evidence to an impartial body.
7. The student has a right to have an adequate and accurate record of the proceedings.

---

It is also important to have policies for dangerous, reckless, or unsafe behaviors to ensure that the clinical nurse educator and academic institution can (a) intervene immediately on behalf of a patient maintaining patient safety and (b) remove the student from the clinical learning environment (CLE) as necessary. A sample policy on unsafe practice is presented in Exhibit 5.2.

---

**Exhibit 5.2  Example of a Policy about Unsafe Behavior**

1. The nursing faculty has an academic, legal, and ethical responsibility to prepare a graduate who is competent as well as to protect the public and healthcare community from unsafe nursing practice. It is within this context that a student may be disciplined or dismissed from the nursing program for practice or behavior that threatens or has the potential to threaten the safety of a patient, a family member or substitute familial person, another student, a faculty member, or other healthcare provider.

2. Every student is expected to be familiar with the principles of safe practice and is expected to perform in accordance with these requirements. Within courses, counseling and advising processes, and other instructional forums, students will be provided with the opportunity to discuss the policy and its implications. Being unprepared for clinical may constitute an unsafe practice and the student may be sent home at the discretion of the clinical nurse educator.

   An *unsafe practice* is defined as the following:

   a. An act or behavior of the type that violates state board of nursing standards of nursing conduct.
   b. An act or behavior of the type that violates the *Code of Ethics* of the American Nurses Association.
   c. An act or behavior that threatens or has the potential to threaten the physical, emotional, mental, or environmental safety of the patient, a family member or substitute familial person, another student, a faculty member, or other healthcare provider (e.g., lack of sleep, medication side effects, substance abuse, or mental or physical conditions; *Duquesne University School of Nursing Student Handbook*, 2017, p. 64).

---

In the event of an incident of unsafe practice, the clinical nurse educator would notify the professional nurse caring for the patient, complete the necessary agency incident report, document the student behavior/incident on the student evaluation form, and notify the course faculty member. Depending on the severity of the incident and pending an internal investigation, the school of nursing could suspend the student. The student would receive the appropriate sanction for the reckless or unsafe behavior, which may include dismissal (Anselmi, Gambescia, & Glasgow, 2014; Duquesne University School of Nursing Student Handbook, 2017; Penn, 2014).

The courts also distinguish between academic dismissals and disciplinary dismissals. They require more due process in disciplinary matters than in academic ones. Although the line is not always clear, it is important to properly classify whether the issue in question is an academic or a disciplinary one. Academic matters in clinical nursing education include the following:

- Matters of personal hygiene, interpersonal skills, and attendance
- Repeated failure to provide clinical assignments
- Inability to handle stress, make sound judgments, and set priorities
- Incompetent clinical performance because of absences or unethical conduct
- Turning in assignments late
- Exhibiting behavior that causes concern such as uncontrolled anger (Smith et al., 2012)

The clinical nurse educator should regard these behaviors as academic in nature and would consider them when evaluating clinical performance. In general, the university conduct board would not be required to deliberate on these behaviors; instead, the clinical nurse educator or academic program should address these behaviors.

The role of the clinical nurse educator encompasses being familiar with the academic and clinical policies at one's institution, providing due process, consulting the department chair or university attorney depending on one's role, documenting events in a timely and objective manner, and following one's institutional policies. Exhibit 5.3 describes critical elements to consider when providing students with due process.

| Exhibit 5.3    Critical Elements to Consider for Due Process |
| --- |
| As a clinical nurse educator, you must provide the student with an opportunity to be heard before rushing to summary judgment. |
| As a clinical nurse educator, you must consult academic policies related to clinical failure prior to informing the student verbally or in writing. |
| If you are a novice clinical nurse educator, ask an experienced faculty member to review your documentation. |
| If you are an experienced faculty member or academic administrator, educate new clinical nurse educators about students' due process rights. |
| Provide the student with advanced notice of a clinical failure. |
| Maintain daily evidence-based anecdotal documentation. |
| Document student behavior in an objective manner, including date, time, location, witnesses, and action taken. |

According to Smith et al. (2012), "most cases related to clinical misconduct or performance issues have been upheld by the courts as long as due process has been afforded to the student and the nursing program followed its own policies" (p. 76).

## ETHICAL DEVELOPMENT IN THE CLINICAL SETTING

The formation of an ethical framework for practice is an essential aspect of nursing students' development and ability to engage in professional nursing practice. Students learn how to apply theory to specific cases and to use *moral reasoning* to establish justified ethical stances about what a student *should do*. The clinical nurse educator's role with respect to ethical development is to serve as a role model and instill moral character in students (Koharchik, Vogelstein, Crider, Devido, & Evatt, 2017). The clinical nurse educator serves as a role model by demonstrating professional behaviors; advocating for the patient's health and welfare, especially in difficult circumstances; reporting reckless behaviors; and acknowledging errors. According to Benner, Sutphen, Leonard-Kahn, and Day (2008), "patient advocacy is alive and well in the everyday ethical aspirations of the student nurses" (p. 474). Formal ethics coursework is essential for students to apply ethics to the clinical environment. The clinical nurse educator is critical to helping students to appreciate the nature of ethically challenging situations and for placing these challenges in the appropriate ethical context (Krautscheid, 2017). Foundational knowledge of ethical theories and practical ethics and proficiency in therapeutic communication are vital to students' understanding of the ethical dilemmas they encounter and avoiding moral distress.

## SUMMARY

The role of the clinical nurse educator is demanding: He or she must balance the learning needs of students and communication needs of nursing staff, keep up to date with clinical knowledge and skills, be familiar with clinical agency and academic nursing programs' policies, and foster ethical development in students (Oermann, 2016). The unique role of the clinical nurse educator requires attentiveness to school/nursing education and clinical practice policies and practices. Research and practice articles focused on the relevant issues pertaining to this positon are needed to build evidence for the clinical nurse educator role.

| 5.1 Clinical Nurse Educator Teaching Tip |
|---|
| The *American Journal of Nursing* (*AJN*) Teaching for Practice column is dedicated to the needs of clinical nurse educators. The *AJN* column offers guidance to the clinical nurse educator on contemporary topics relevant in clinical nursing education. |

### 5.1 Case Study

**Clinical Nurse Educator in an Accelerated BSN Program**

Dr. Molloy is the clinical nurse educator on a medical–surgical unit for BSN second-degree students in a 12-month accelerated program. She observes that Sasha Gosherova looks very tired. As her clinical instructor, Sasha informed Dr. Molloy that she would be late for clinical due to her work schedule. She tells Dr. Molloy that she needs to work and does not have family in this country to support her. Dr. Molloy also learns that Ms. Gosherova commutes 2 hours a day in addition to working full-time nights as a PCT and is attending the second-degree accelerated BSN program full time. Dr. Molloy calculates that Sasha is awake at least 20 hours per day due to her class and work schedule and commuting time.

**Questions for Reflection:**

How do nurse educators develop policies for students while taking into account students' needs?

How would a clinical nurse educator monitor a work policy?

What student behaviors would alert a clinical nurse educator to question whether the student is violating the work policy?

**Case Analysis**

After observing the student and hearing the student's account of her work schedule and obligations, Dr. Molloy informs Sasha that she needs to report to the clinical environment on time as per the clinical objectives and as is expected of her student colleagues. Dr. Malloy refers Sasha to the assistant dean for Student Affairs to inquire about additional financial aid. Dr. Molloy also consults the course faculty member/coordinator about the existence of any academic policies on sleep requirements and consecutive working hours or unsafe practice. Dr. Molloy also consults with the clinical agency about a policy on sleep requirements and consecutive nursing hours for professional nurses to determine whether a nurse is limited on the number of consecutive hours he or she can work in a 24-hour period. After consultation, Dr. Molloy learns that the university has a policy on student employment that references sleep (refer to student employment policy), and the clinical agency has a policy on consecutive nursing hours worked, limiting nurses generally to 12.5 hours of work in a 24-hour period. Sasha is informed in writing that she cannot work *and* go to school more than 12.5 hours per each 24-hour period and needs to obtain adequate sleep to be a safe clinician. Failure to comply will result in disciplinary action. See the example of a student employment policy for clinical practice (Exhibit 5.4).

PCT, patient care technician.

### Exhibit 5.4 Student Employment Policy

- School of nursing will not accommodate work schedules for course registration or clinical placement. In addition, students are not permitted to work overnight/night shift prior to attending clinical as this practice is unsafe for the student and patient(s). If a student is found to have worked overnight prior to attending clinical, he or she will face disciplinary sanctions.

- Second-degree students are strongly discouraged from working during the 12-month second-degree BSN program due to the academic rigor and intensity of the program (*Duquesne University School of Nursing Student Handbook*, 2017, p. 20).

Student nurses can be held liable for their actions and can be sued. A student nurse is held to the same standard of care as an RN when performing RN duties. If a student nurse cannot safely function in the performance of these duties while unsupervised, the student should not be carrying out RN duties. In another set of circumstances in which a clinical nurse educator is present, the clinical nurse educator might have been found liable had the clinical nurse educator knowingly allowed the student to care for patients with very limited or no sleep (Paterson & Lane, 2000; Smith et al., 2012).

## ▦ REVIEW QUESTIONS

1. The clinical nurse educator is conducting preconference and a junior nursing student is unable to answer questions about her assigned patient's diagnosis or safety concerns. The clinical nurse educator should:

   A. Send the student off the clinical unit.

   B. Coassign the student to another student nurse.

   C. Assign the student to a nurse.

   D. Issue a clinical failure for the course.

2. The clinical nurse educator learns that a student in her clinical group is working a full-time night shift and going to an accelerated nursing program full time. The clinical nurse educator should:

   A. Do nothing as the student's work schedule is not the school's concern.

   B. Inform the student in writing that she needs to follow the policy related to consecutive nursing hours.

   C. Allow the student to begin clinical at a later time.

   D. Call the student's employer.

3. The clinical nurse educator issues a learning contract to her nursing student for which purpose?

   A. In order to award a clinical warning

   B. To protect the faculty against litigation

   C. To assist student in meeting the clinical objectives

   D. In order to award a failing grade

4. The focus of the remediation plan should be to:

   A. Support student learning and mastery of competencies.

   B. Document clinical deficiencies.

   C. Protect the faculty member against litigation.

   D. Acknowledge students' clinical competence.

5. Due process, as it applies to clinical nursing education, is described as:

   A. Procedural safeguards that are established in protection of patient safety.

   B. Procedural safeguards that are established in protection of academic honesty.

   C. Procedural safeguards that are established in protection of student privacy.

   D. Procedural safeguards that are established based on how issues of academic misconduct or performance will be treated.

6. "Just culture" applied to clinical nursing education is described as:

   A. Critical incident debriefing is held with the nursing staff.

   B. Students learn and improve by openly identifying and examining their weaknesses.

   C. Students attend all required remediation sessions.

   D. Students can question the clinical nurse educator.

7. Reckless behavior for students engaged in a clinical practicum would include:

   A. Arriving late to clinical

   B. Reporting positive information to the clinical nurse educator

   C. Failing to follow the chain of command

   D. Lack of clinical preparation

8. A student misreads a medication label on a busy medical–surgical floor resulting in a near-miss medication error. This type of error is described as:

   A. Human error

   B. At-risk error

   C. Reckless error

   D. Rule-based error

9. If a nursing student engages in abusive, bullying behaviors, the clinical educator would consider this behavior as:

   A. Lapsed behavior

   B. At-risk behavior

   C. Reckless behavior

   D. Skill-based behavior

10. If a student looks up or discusses private information about patients outside of specified patient assignment/responsibilities, this behavior would be considered:

    A. Human error

    B. At-risk behavior

    C. Reckless behavior

    D. Knowledge-based behavior

## ▦ REFERENCES

Andrew, S., Halcomb, E. J., Jackson, D., Peters, K., & Salamonson, Y. (2010). Sessional teachers in a BN program: Bridging the divide or widening the gap. *Nurse Education Today, 30*(5), 453–457. doi:10.1016/j.nedt.2009.10.004

Anselmi, K. L., Gambescia, S., & Smith Glasgow, M. E. (2014). Using a student conduct committee to foster professional accountability. *Journal of Professional Nursing, 30*(6), 481–485. doi:10.1016/j.profnurs.2014.04.002

Barnsteiner, J., & Disch, J. (2017a). Creating a fair and just culture in schools of nursing. *American Journal of Nursing, 117*(11), 42–48. doi:10.1097/01.NAJ.0000526747.84173.97

Barnsteiner, J., & Disch, J. (2017b). Exploring how nursing schools handle student errors and near misses. *American Journal of Nursing, 117*(10), 24–31. doi:10.1097/01.NAJ.0000525849.35536.74

Benner, P., Sutphen, M., Leonard-Kahn, V., & Day, L. (2008). Formation and everyday ethical comportment. *American Journal of Critical Care, 17*(5), 473–476.

Boysen, P. (2013). Just culture: A foundation for balanced accountability and patient safety. *Ochsner Journal, 13*(3), 400–406.

Brown, Y., Neudorf, K., Poitras, C., & Rodger, K. (2007). Unsafe clinical performance calls for a systematic approach. *Canadian Nurse, 103*(3), 29–32.

Dekker, S. (2008). *Just culture: Balancing safety and accountability.* Burlington, VT: Ashgate.

Duquesne University School of Nursing Student Handbook. (2017). *Traditional BSN and second degree student handbook, 2017–2018 academic year.* Retrieved from https://www.duq.edu/assets/Documents/nursing/Handbooks/Duquesne-SON-UG-handbook-2017-18.pdf

Gardner, M. R., & Suplee, P. D. (2010). *Handbook of clinical teaching in nursing and health sciences.* Sudbury, MA: Jones & Bartlett.

Johnson, E. G. (2009). The academic performance of students: Legal and ethical issues. In D. M. Billings & J. A. Halstead, *Teaching in nursing: A guide for faculty* (pp. 33–52). St. Louis, MO: Saunders.

Kaplin, W. A., & Lee, B. A. (2013). *The law of higher education* (5th ed.). San Francisco, CA: Jossey-Bass.

Koharchik, L., Vogelstein, E., Crider, M., Devido, J., & Evatt, M. (2017). Promoting nursing student's ethical development in the clinical setting. *American Journal of Nursing, 117*(11), 57–60. doi:10.1097/01.NAJ.0000526750.07045.79

Kolanko, K., Clark, C., Heinrich, K., Olive, D., Serembus, J., & Sifford, K. (2006). Academic dishonesty, bullying, incivility, and violence: Difficult challenges facing nurse educators. *Nursing Education Perspectives, 27*(1), 34–43.

Krautscheid, L. C. (2017). Embedding microethical dilemmas in high fidelity simulation scenarios: Preparing nursing students for ethical practice. *Journal of Nursing Education, 56*(1), 55–58. doi:10.3928/01484834-20161219-11

Lindsay, C. L. III. (2005). *The college student's guide to the law.* Dallas, TX: Taylor Trade.

Marx, D. (2001). *Patient safety and the "just culture": A primer for health care executives.* New York, NY: Trustees of Columbia University.

McGregor, A. (2007). Academic success, clinical failure: Struggling practices of a failing student. *Journal of Nursing Education, 46*(11), 504–511.

Oermann, M. H. (2016). Reflections on clinical teaching in nursing. *Nurse Educator, 41*(4), 165. doi:10.1097/NNE.0000000000000279

Paterson, C., & Lane, L. (2000). An analysis of legal issues concerning university-based nursing education programs. *Journal of Nursing Law, 7*(2), 7–18.

Patton, C. W., & Lewallen, L. P. (2015). Legal issues in clinical nursing education. *Nurse Educator, 40*(3), 124–128. doi:10.1097/NNE.0000000000000122

Penn, C. (2014). Integrating just culture into nursing student error policy. *Journal of Nursing Education, 53*(9), S107–S109. doi:10.3928/01484834-20140806-02

Reason, J. (1997). *Managing the risks of organizational accidents.* Burlington, VT: Ashgate.

Roth, J. (2007). *Higher education law in America* (8th ed.). Malvern, PA: Center for Education and Employment Law.

Santisteban, L., & Egues, A. L. (2014). Cultivating adjunct faculty: Strategies beyond orientation. *Nursing Forum, 49*(3), 152–158. doi:10.1111/nuf.12106

Smith, M. H., McKoy, E., & Richardson, J. (2001). Legal issues related to dismissing students for clinical deficiencies. *Nurse Educator, 26*(1), 33–38. doi:10.1097/00006223-200101000-00015

Smith Glasgow, M. E., & Dreher, H. M. (2007). Legal issues in student supervision. *Advance for Nursing, 9*(18), 37–41.

Smith Glasgow, M. E., Dreher, H. M., & Oxholm, C. (2012). *Legal issues confronting today's nursing faculty: A case-study approach.* Philadelphia, PA: F. A. Davis.

Strader, M. K. (1985). Malpractice and nurse educators: Defining legal responsibilities. *Journal of Nursing Education, 24*(9), 363–367. doi:10.3928/0148-4834-19851101-06

Suplee, P. D., & Gardner, M. (2009). Fostering a smooth transition to the faculty role. *Journal of Continuing Education in Nursing, 40*(11), 514–520. doi:10.3928/00220124-20091023-09

Suplee, P. D., Lachman, V., Seibert, B., & Anselmi, K. (2008). Managing nursing incivility in the classroom, clinical setting, and on-line. *Journal of Nursing Law, 12*(2), 68–77. doi:10.1891/1073-7472.12.2.68

Whitney, K. M. (2009). Managing the learning environment: Proactively responding to student misconduct. In D. M. Billings & J. A. Halstead, *Teaching in nursing: A guide for faculty* (pp. 227–237). St. Louis, MO: Saunders.

# 6

# Facilitate Learning in the Healthcare Environment

*M. ANNIE MULLER*

*In the middle of every difficulty lies opportunity.*
—Albert Einstein

## ▧ LEARNING OUTCOMES

At the end of this chapter, the learner will be able to

- Recognize special needs of the culturally diverse student.
- Incorporate ethics in healthcare through interprofessional collaboration.
- Improve competencies through mentorship.
- Improve collegial collaboration in the clinical setting.

## ▧ INTRODUCTION

Facilitating learning for the student in the clinical learning environment (CLE) is only one aspect of nursing education. Clinical practice is the larger part of nursing education and it is essential that the clinical nurse educator be competent and well prepared in her or his knowledge and skills (Preethy, Erna, & Mariamma, 2014). Learning in the CLE can enhance skills learned in the lab as well as provide for integration of the application of theory learned in the classrooms (Hutchinson & Goodwin, 2013). Based on the NLN's *Certified Academic Clinical Nurse Educator (CNE®cl) 2018 Candidate Handbook* (National League for Nursing [NLN], 2018), there are eight task statements that will guide the nurse educator toward facilitating learning in the healthcare environment.

## ▓ IMPLEMENTING A VARIETY OF TEACHING STRATEGIES

Research shows clinical placement of students should offer best practices as well as multiple opportunities that will influence their learning outcomes. The CLE can have a positive or negative effect on the students' professional development based on the reception from the staff during a clinical rotation. Therefore, the skill, communication, and engagement of the clinical nurse educator are important to ensure the CLE is positive. Clinical nurse educators use a variety of teaching strategies in order to assist students to bridge the theory–practice gap. Literature regarding teaching strategies in the CLE reveals the following:

- Nurse educators who use active learning strategies in the CLE allow the students to develop specialized skills such as critical thinking, prioritizing, communicating, and collaborating with other professionals (Moyer, 2016).

- In the CLE, the student needs to be able to use both the theory learned in class as well as the skills learned in the lab (Papastavrou, Dimitriadou, Tsangari, & Andreou, 2016).

- Many different methods were found to facilitate teaching strategies; however, they all had one main theme: to involve the student in active learning and engagement (Staykova, Stewart, & Staykov, 2017).

- By incorporating both theory and evidence-based practice for students, the clinical educator needs to consider the student population, especially those students who may come from another country. The international student needs to have special teaching considerations to understand the culture of the population in which she or he learns (Mikkonen, Elo, Kuivila, Tuomikoski, & Kaariainen, 2016).

## ▓ GROUNDING TEACHING STRATEGIES

Evidence-based teaching practices are developing for both the classroom and the CLE.

Five areas that emphasizes the need for further development of evidence-based teaching practices (Kalb, O'Connor-Von, Brockway, Rierson, & Sendelbach, 2015) are the following:

- Curriculum teaching
- Learning and evaluation strategies
- Resources
- Innovation
- Educational research

| 6.1 Evidence-Based Clinical Teaching Practice |
| --- |
| A study done by Staykova et al. (2017) describes the need for both traditional and new strategies to improve and facilitate learning, especially when teaching the adult learner. The adult is more apt to engage in active learning when faculty use strategies to transition from passive learning in the classroom to active learning in the clinical setting. |

Examples of evidence-based teaching strategies are summarized in Table 6.1.

| Table 6.1 Examples of Teaching Strategies and Descriptions | |
| --- | --- |
| Traditional didactic | Traditional didactic teaching can be done in the classroom or the laboratory; it focuses on preparing for examinations or specific skills. PowerPoint, lecture, exams, quizzes, and discussions are examples of tools used in traditional didactic learning. |
| Evidence-based case scenarios | Presentations of current research or evidence-based situations allow the students to role-play and use critical thinking to problem-solve situations in a controlled environment. |
| Admission tickets | Use of admission tickets allows the faculty to have students complete preclass assignments for a planned experience in the skills lab. Students need to review material, view a training video, or complete exercises to be familiar with lab expectations and be prepared to perform said skill in the lab. |
| I-clicker | This is an audience response system frequently used during lectures, which involves active learning by allowing the student to select answers to questions posed in class. This promotes discussion on lecture content. |
| Gaming | This is used to promote understanding of key concepts of the lecture, developing cognitive skills in both the didactic and lab setting. |
| Simulation | Creating a real-life setting in a controlled environment allows the student to experience the role of a nurse. The controlled setting allows any error that occurs to be corrected without harm to anyone. In addition, once the simulation has been completed a debriefing is conducted in which all events are discussed. |

*Source:* Staykova, M. P., Stewart, D. V., & Staykov, D. I. (2017). Back to basics and beyond: Comparing traditional and innovative strategies for teaching in nursing skills laboratories. *Teaching and Learning in Nursing, 12,* 152–157. doi: 10.1016/j.teln.2016.12.0.

## ▓ CREATING OPPORTUNITIES

*Critical thinking* can be defined in many different ways, one of which is the ability to process information, problem-solve, and purposefully self-regulate judgment, which results in interpretation, analysis, evaluation, and the ability to make inferences (Macauley, Brudvig, Kadakia, & Bonneville, 2017; Pitt, Powis, Levett-Jones, & Hunter, 2015).

- One method of teaching critical thinking is to incorporate case-based assignments into the curriculum (Heath & Weege, 2017) using:
  - ▧ Simulation
  - ▧ Real-life situations/scenarios
  - ▧ Role-play
- In a study by Raymond, Profetto-McGrath, Myrick, and Stream (2018), application of nursing theoretical knowledge in practice facilitated the development of the nursing students' critical thinking skills.
- The clinical nurse educator had a strong impact in the role of teaching critical thinking to students based on the educator's experience and interactions with the students (Raymond et al., 2018).
- Educational strategies that promote critical thinking can include reflective journaling. As a pedagogical strategy, the structuring of the journal assignment reflects an analytical framework by using a case scenario to focus on specific elements (Webster, 2018).

---

**6.1 Clinical Nurse Educator Teaching Tip**

Often, multiple nursing schools use a clinical facility and each of which has different expectations of what their students should be learning during their clinical rotation. In addition, the students will have different levels of knowledge based on their level in school. Therefore, when bringing a group of students to the clinical site, it is a good idea to have a list of expectations of the clinical student to give to the unit nurses and staff. This document should be posted in each nursing station and outline specific details such as

- Specific student objectives
- Student names and their patient room assignments
- The students' expected roles and duties for the day, for example:
  - ▧ Medication administration
  - ▧ Specific treatment skills
  - ▧ Being the charge nurse
- Faculty contact information should a need arise

---

## ▧ USING TECHNOLOGY

Expanding healthcare practices are challenging nurse educators to incorporate advanced technology into education and clinical practices (Mackay, Anderson, & Harding, 2017).

- Incorporating technology, such as mobile apps, improves the knowledge base, critical thinking, and clinical competencies of the students (Mackay et al., 2017).
- Mobile apps allow students access to the most current and up-to-date information and improve performance in the clinical setting (Raman, 2015).

- Examples of free mobile apps:
  - ▦ UpToDate is a mobile app that allows the learner to have access to current evidence-based practices in clinical decision-making, medication information, patient education, and links to full-text articles.
  - ▦ Bright Futures is an app that allows the learner to have up-to-date information on disease prevention and health promotion for infants, children, adolescents, and their families.
  - ▦ CDC is an app that allows the learner to see current standards for immunizations required for infants, children, adolescents, teens, and adults. It also offers current information regarding diseases and prevention, including healthy living and safe health tips for travelers.
- Simulation-based learning allows the student to experience scenarios students may not encounter in the clinical setting by interacting with high-fidelity simulators or standardized patients (Raurell-Torreda & Romero-Collado, 2015).
- Interprofessional healthcare-simulation–based learning offers students the opportunity to collaborate with other healthcare professionals (Craig, McInroy, Bogo, & Thompson, 2017).

## ▦ PROMOTE A CULTURE OF SAFETY AND QUALITY IN THE HEALTHCARE ENVIRONMENT

- The Quality and Safety Education for Nurses (QSEN) initiative established five mandates for nursing students, with safety first on the list (Cooper, 2013).
- The QSEN framework was established to clearly outline what competencies are expected of nursing students (Cooper, 2013).
- Shortages of nursing educators, nursing students, and nurses create a crisis, which underscores the need to maintain safety in the healthcare environment (Mundt, Clark, & Klemczak, 2013).
- Poor communication between staff and providers creates a hazardous situation that leads to an unsafe environment (Mundt et al., 2013).
- Medication administration is a part of patient care and medication errors most likely occur more often than reported (Vaismoradi, Jordan, Turunen, & Bondas, 2014).
- Reasons for not reporting medication errors (Vaismoradi et al., 2014) include:
  - ▦ Fear of managers
  - ▦ Fear of losing job
  - ▦ Fear of legal implications
  - ▦ Fear and embarrassment in the presence of peers

- Other safety issues to consider (Mundt et al., 2013) are the following:
  - ▓ Increased patient acuity in the hospital setting
  - ▓ Shorter lengths of stay for illnesses
  - ▓ Increased stress on nurses

A *Quality and Safety Officer (QSO)* position was created at one university to promote safety and quality care in the CLE among students (Cooper, 2013). In addition to the facility-required reports, QSOs developed two new reports for the nursing students:

- Formal error report
- Near-miss report

A *root cause analysis,* which is a method of problem-solving to get to the source of the issue, is useful in establishing open lines of communication between faculty and student (Cooper, 2013).

## ■ CREATING A POSITIVE LEARNING ENVIRONMENT

Students who are intimidated by their clinical nurse educators become anxious, which impedes their ability to apply knowledge learned in the classroom to the clinical setting (Hutchinson & Goodwin, 2013; Moscaritolo, 2009). Table 6.2 describes methods to reduce students' anxiety.

| Table 6.2 Methods to Reduce Student Anxiety | |
| --- | --- |
| Faculty–student interactions | Caring transactions are a meaningful way for faculty to engage in dialogue with a student and promote critical thinking. |
| Teach mindfulness | Mindfulness is an intervention that helps decrease anxiety through breathing, meditation, walking, and self-reflection. |
| Use of humor | Humor reduces anxiety and stress, makes learning fun, focuses students' attention, strengthens social relationships, increases self-esteem, and improves performance. |

The attitude of the clinical nurse educator has a positive or negative effect on students, especially those who differ culturally and linguistically from other students. Negative attitudes tend to impede students from learning to have caring feelings (Mikkonen et al., 2016). Working in an atmosphere where they feel appreciated and accepted has a positive impact on student learning outcomes (Bisholt, Ohlsson, Engstrom, Johansson, & Gustafsson, 2014).

Characteristics that promote a good working environment for students are (Bisholt et al., 2014):

- Staff attitude
- Supervisory relationship
- Leadership style
- Quality of care provided
- Cooperation between healthcare facility and the nursing school

As mentioned, students from different cultures may have additional learning and socialization needs. Positive learning experiences for students were enhanced when an intercultural mentor was present in the clinical setting (Mikkonen, Elo, Tuomikoski, & Kaariainen, 2016).

---

**6.2   Clinical Nurse Educator Teaching Tip**

At the end of the semester or clinical rotation, it is important for the students to sign a *thank-you* card for the nurses and staff. The nurses and staff work hard and many take extra time to teach the students' knowledge and skills they otherwise may not see until after being employed at a healthcare facility. Having the students acknowledge the work and knowledge shared by the nurses and staff builds goodwill with the school, the facility, and the clinical nurse educator, and improves collegial work for the future.

---

## ▓ DEVELOPING COLLEGIAL WORKING RELATIONSHIPS

Collaboration between schools of nursing and healthcare agencies fosters an increase in goodwill between the agencies and nursing academia in practice (Mager & Bradley, 2013).

Collaborative models used between healthcare organizations and educational institutions are innovative and produce positive outcomes for both entities. Examples of collaborative models (American Association of Colleges of Nursing [AACN], 2002, 2019); Mager & Bradley, 2013) are listed in Table 6.3.

**Table 6.3  Collaborative Methods**

| Collaborative Model | Program Highlights | Collaborative School |
|---|---|---|
| Clinical Scholar | Clinical appointment made by university for expert staff in a variety of settings | University of Colorado |
| Cooperative Education Program | Hospital staff RN and student work together on the same shift and schedule; staff RN contributes to student's evaluation | University of Alabama |
| Partnership for Advancing Home Care Education and Practice | Home healthcare agency collaborates with university to provide access to clinical sites and clinical teaching; both university and home health agency have equal representation on the advisory board | Simmons College |

*Source:* American Association of Colleges of Nursing. (2002). *Using strategic partnerships to expand nursing education programs; Successful partner profiles.* Washington, DC: Author. American Association of Colleges of Nursing. (2019). *Academic-practice partnerships tool kit.* Retrieved from https://www.aacnnursing.org/Academic-Practice-Partnerships/Implementation-Tool-Kit

> ### 6.2 Evidence-Based Clinical Teaching Practice
>
> A study done by Stout, Short, Aldrich, Cintron, and Provencio-Vasquez (2015) demonstrated the success of a new internship/nurse residency program. As part of the IOM recommendations, a new-nurse residency program was established in a town in Texas. The outcomes of the study showed the costs associated with the program were outweighed by its effects as the quality of care improved, fewer medication errors occurred, and new-nurse retention increased.
>
> IOM, Institute of Medicine.

> ### 6.3 Evidence-Based Clinical Teaching Practice
>
> A study by Pearson, Wyte-Lake, Bowman, Needleman, and Dobalian (2015) showed that having students partner with staff nurses increased the clinical education activities designed to foster evidence-based practices on the unit.

Part of establishing partnerships is cultivating positive relationships. Relationships improved between faculty and nursing staff when the staff was made aware of the nursing programs goals; this, in turn, increased staff satisfaction when working with the students and faculty and decreased feelings of being burdened with students. A strategy to create a practice partnership discussed by Wonder and York (2017) is to have learning activities for students that help the staff nurses develop evidence-based polices used in the clinical setting.

- Faculty, students, and clinical leaders collaborate during policy reviews to update outdated polices with more current evidence-based practices (Wonder & York, 2017).

- Assign a team of members who work collaboratively to work on one policy that demonstrates how this new policy improves and enhances nursing knowledge and skills and present this information to the administration (Wonder & York, 2017).

## ▦ DEMONSTRATING ENTHUSIASM FOR TEACHING

- Traditional teaching may not reach the millennial learners of today, who are technologically savvy (Ebert, 2016). Young and Seibenhener (2018) discuss students' need for a new, more diverse way of teaching and note the following:

  - Students are more concerned with recording information than listening and learning.

  - Visual, aural, or kinesthetic students need a different method of information presentation to accommodate their learning styles.

  - Identify the learning style of the student to meet the learning outcomes (learning styles are discussed in Chapter 2, Test-Taking Strategies, and Chapter 9, Facilitate Learner Development and Socialization).

- A study done by Johnson and Barrett (2017) discusses autonomous active learning. This is considered more effective than passive learning.
  - ■ Active learning is a pedagogical practice
    - Educators facilitate and empower the students
    - Students become owners of their own learning and education, taking responsibility for engaging in what they learn
  - ■ Strategies to help motivate students to learn:
    - Games, such as answering *Jeopardy*-style questions
    - Quiz bowl, in which groups determine the correct answer to questions

## ■ SUMMARY

The clinical nurse educators' role to facilitate learning in the healthcare environment involves an ever-changing process. The innovations of new technology, student learning needs, and staying current with evidence-based practice challenge the nurse educator to constantly be aware of such changes. The clinical nurse educator will need to be accommodating and adapt to change to be able to bring new ideas from the classroom to promote and enhance student learning. Implementing new ideas in the CLE improves the success of the student who may have a different style of learning. Adding interest in the CLE greatly enhances the desire for the nursing student to learn new concepts and increases critical thinking skills. In order for the clinical nurse educator to meet the IOM (2010) goals to develop a more highly educated workforce, clinical nurse educators need to take an active role in the lifelong learning process. Although change is not always a welcomed event, change needs to happen for clinical nurse educators to continue to grow and to meet the demanding needs of the students, faculty, and community.

---

**6.1 Case Study**

The clinical nurse educator for a group of first-semester nursing students was working with a student assigned to administer medications to a selected patient. Once the student researched all medications to be given at the assigned time, the clinical nurse educator and the student reviewed each medication per the objectives of the class. The student was tasked with knowing about the drug classifications, its intended use, side effects, and the basic five rights of medication administration. When the student began to retrieve the medications from the medication cabinet, using the MAR, the clinical nurse educator noticed the student was retrieving medications for a patient other than the one who had been assigned. The assigned patient and the patient the student was pulling meds for had very similar first names and the same last names. The clinical nurse educator cautioned the student to be sure to check the names again, after which the student still believed she was pulling meds for the correct patient. Once the student was at the patient's door, the clinical nurse educator again asked the student to verify the correct assigned patient with the MAR, and again, the

---

*(continued)*

---

**6.1 Case Study (*continued*)**

student believed she had the correct patient. For the final check, the clinical nurse educator had the student check the ID band for the patient against the MAR and finally the student realized she had the wrong medication for her patient. The clinical nurse educator asked to speak with the student outside of the patient's room to debrief what had just occurred. In a private room, the clinical nurse educator and student discussed in detail what had occurred and why after being asked to verify the correct patient three times, did the student not see the medication was for the incorrect patient. The student was completely devastated by the possibility that a medication error could have occurred if she had been less vigilant. The student never made this mistake again as she progressed through the program.

**Questions for Reflection:**

1. What should have the clinical nurse educator done differently?

2. Prior to standing before the patient's door, could the clinical nurse educator have explained about the error that was about to occur?

3. How would you have handled the student in a similar situation?

MAR, medication administration record.

---

## ▦ REVIEW QUESTIONS

1. Clinical nurse educators should consider using various methods of teaching. According to visual, aural/auditory, read/write, and kinesthetic (VARK) learners, which learning style enjoys listening to tape recordings and problem-solving?

   A. Visual learners

   B. Kinesthetic learners

   C. Multimodal learners

   D. Audio learners

2. To meet the learning needs of the student, the nurse educator will need to develop several strategies for teaching. Which of the following strategies would best demonstrate the model of education that meets the needs of the student?

   A. Student centered

   B. Group centered

   C. Nursing centered

   D. Educator centered

3. The nurse educator is collecting data to analyze information that can improve instruction and student learning while it is happening. Which of the following best explains this type of assessment?

   A. Summative assessment

   B. Formative assessment

   C. Diagnostic assessment

   D. Impact assessment

4. The nursing faculty and administration plan to make a major change in the curriculum for the nursing program. The department realizes the current status quo will be destabilized. According to Lewin's theory of change, which stage of change would be occurring at this time?

A. Unfreezing

B. Movement

C. Refreezing

D. Debriefing

5. Which of the following could be considered a nursing theory that promotes and helps the student become self-sufficient?

A. Self-care

B. Self-aware

C. Autocratic

D. Reliant

6. In the quality improvement of education, which of the following would the clinical nurse educator include in the clinical experiences?

A. Best evidence

B. Past experiences

C. Recent events

D. Local customs

7. Nursing turnover can be very costly to the administration. One way to reduce that turnover is to provide nursing mentors. Which of the following best demonstrates the purpose and end result of having a nursing mentor?

A. A retention strategy

B. A relationship builder

C. A best friend

D. A career guide

8. Clinical evaluations and assessment data are kept for many reasons. Which of the following explains the best reason for keeping these data?

A. They help to determine the achievement of the student.

B. They encourage the students' progress in the course.

C. They allow others to see how a great educational program is taught.

D. They emphasize the experience the clinical nurse educator demonstrates.

9. The nursing department is advertising for a clinical nurse educator to help redesign the clinical component of the curriculum. Which of the following type of clinical nurse educator would have the skills to create and articulate a positive change?

A. Someone with good people skills

B. Someone with very high personal integrity

C. Someone with a great strategic vision

D. Someone with excellent technical skills

**10.** The clinical nurse educator is evaluating a student who is having difficulty understanding basic concepts presented in the clinical learning environment. Which of the following would be the first step the nurse educator should take to help this student?

A. Enroll the student in a remediation course.

B. Send the student to the student learning center for evaluation.

C. Have the student take a visual, aural/auditory, read/write, and kinesthetic (VARK) test to see what learning style the student has.

D. Have the student study with a group of senior students.

# ▨ REFERENCES

American Association of Colleges of Nursing. (2002). *Using strategic partnerships to expand nursing education programs: Successful partner profiles.* Washington, DC: Author.

American Association of Colleges of Nursing. (2019). *Academic-practice partnerships tool kit.* Retrieved from https://www.aacnnursing.org/Academic-Practice-Partnerships/Implementation-Tool-Kit

Bisholt, B., Ohlsson, U., Engstrom, A. K., Johansson, A. S., & Gustafsson, M. (2014). Nursing students' assessment of the learning environment in different clinical settings. *Nurse Educator in Practice, 14,* 304–310. doi:10.1016/j.nepr.2013.11.005

Cooper, E. (2013). From the school of nursing quality and safety officer: Nursing students' use of safety reporting tools and their perception of safety issues in clinical settings. *Journal of Professional Nursing, 29*(2), 109–116. doi:10.1016/j.profnurs.2012.12.005

Craig, S. L., McInroy, L. B., Bogo, M., & Thompson, M. (2017). Enhancing competence in health social work education through simulation based learning: Strategies from a case study of a family session. *Journal of Social Work Education, 53*(1), 547–558. doi:10.1080/10437797.2017.1288597

Ebert, K. (2016). Teaching techniques: Classroom strategies for millennial learners. *Radiation Therapist, 25*(2), 201–204.

Heath, A., & Weege, M. (2017). Improving critical thinking through case-based lectures. *Radiation Therapist, 26*(2), 206–208.

Hutchinson, T. L., & Goodwin, H. J. (2013). Nursing student anxiety as context for teaching/learning. *Journal of Holistic Nursing, 3*(1), 19–24. doi:10.1177/0898010112462067

Institute of Medicine of the National Academies. (2010). *The future of nursing: Focus on education.* Washington, DC: National Academies Press. Retrieved from http://www.nationalacademies.org/hmd/~/media/Files/Report%20Files/2010/The-Future-of-Nursing/Nursing%20Education%202010%20Brief.pdf

Johnson, H., & Barrett, L. C. (2017). Your teaching strategy matters: How engagement impacts application in health. *Journal of Medical Library Association, 105*(1), 44–48. doi:10.5195/jmla.2017.8

Kalb, K. A., O'Connor-Von, S. K., Brockway, C., Rierson, C. L., & Sendelbach, S. (2015). Evidence-based teaching practice in nursing education: Faculty perspectives and practice. *Nursing Education Perspective, 36*(4), 212–219. doi:10.5480/14-1472

Macauley, K., Brudvig, T., Kadakia, M., & Bonneville, M. (2017). Systematic review of assessments that evaluate clinical decision making, clinical reasoning, and critical thinking changes after simulation participation. *Journal of Physical Therapy Education, 31*(4), 64–75. doi:10.1097/JTE.0000000000000011

Mackay, B. J., Anderson, J., & Harding, T. (2017). Mobile technology in clinical teaching. *Nurse Education in Practice, 22,* 1–6. doi:10.1016/j.nepr.2016.11.001

Mager, D. R., & Bradley, S. (2013). Collaboration between home healthcare agencies and schools of nursing. *Home Healthcare Nurse, 31*(9), 482–492. doi:10.1097/NHH.0b013e3182a992df

Mikkonen, K., Elo, S., Kuivila, H.-M., Tuomikoski, A.-M., & Kaariainen, M. (2016). Culturally and linguistically diverse healthcare students' experiences of learning in a clinical environment: A systematic review of qualitative studies. *International Journal of Nursing Studies, 54,* 173–187. doi:10.1016/j.ijnurstu.2015.06.004

Mikkonen, K., Elo, S., Tuomikoski, A.-M., & Kaariainen, M. (2016). Mentor experiences of international healthcare students' learning in a clinical environment: A systematic review. *Nurse Education Today, 40,* 87–94. doi:10.1016/j.nedt.2016.02.013

Moscaritolo, L. M. (2009). Interventional strategies to decrease nursing students anxiety in the clinical learning environment. *Journal of Nursing Education, 48*(1), 17–23. doi:10.3928/01484834-20090101-08

Moyer, S. M. (2016). Large group simulation: Using combined teaching strategies to connect classroom and clinical learning. *Teaching and Learning in Nursing, 11*, 67–73. doi:10.1016/j.teln.2016.01.002

Mundt, M. H., Clark, M. P., & Klemczak, J. W. (2013). A task force model for statewide change in nursing education: Building quality and safety. *Journal of Professional Nursing, 29*(2), 117–123. doi:10.1016/j.profnurs.2012.12.008

National League for Nursing. (2018). *Certified academic clinical nurse educator (CNE® cl) 2018 candidate handbook.* Retrieved from http://www.nln.org/docs/default-source/default-document-library/cnecl-handbook-jan-2018.pdf?sfvrsn=4

Papastavrou, E., Dimitriadou, M., Tsangari, H., & Andreou, C. (2016). Nursing students' satisfaction of the clinical learning environment: A research study. *BioMed Central Nursing, 15*(44), 1–10.

Pearson, M. L., Wyte-Lake, T., Bowman, C., Needleman, J., & Dobalian, A. (2015). Assessing the impact of academic-practice partnerships on nursing staff. *BioMed Central Nursing, 14*, 28. doi:10.1186/s12912-015-0085-7

Pitt, V., Powis, D., Levett-Jones, T., & Hunter, S. (2015). The influence of critical thinking skills on performance and progression in the pre-registration nursing program. *Nurse Education Today, 35*(1), 125–131. doi:10.1016/j.nedt.2014.08.006

Preethy, J., Erna, J. R., & Mariamma, V. G. (2014). A comparative study to assess the perception of doctors, nurses, faculty of nursing and nursing students on ideal clinical learning environment. *International Journal of Nursing Education, 6*(1), 208–212. doi:10.5958/j.0974-9357.6.1.042

Raman, J. (2015). Mobile technology in nursing education: Where do we go from here? A review of the literature. *Nurse Education Today, 35*, 663–672. doi:10.1016/j.nedt.2015.01.018

Raurell-Torreda, M., & Romero-Collado, A. (2015). Simulation-based learning as a tactic for teaching evidence-based practice. *Worldviews on Evidence-Based Nursing, 12*(6), 392–394. doi:10.1111/wvn.12107

Raymond, C., Profetto-McGrath, J., Myrick, F., & Stream, W. (2018). Balancing the seen and unseen: Nurse educator as role model for critical thinking. *Nurse Education in Practice, 31*, 41–47. doi:10.1016/j.nepr.2018.04.010

Staykova, M. P., Stewart, D. V., & Staykov, D. I. (2017). Back to basics and beyond: Comparing traditional and innovative strategies for teaching in nursing skills laboratories. *Teaching and Learning in Nursing, 12*, 152–157. doi: 10.1016/j.teln.2016.12.001

Stout, C., Short, N., Aldrich, K., Cintron, R. J., & Provencio-Vasquez, E. (2015). Meeting the Future of Nursing Report™ recommendations: A successful practice-academic partnership. *Nursing Economics, 33*(3), 161–166.

Vaismoradi, M., Jordan, S., Turunen, H., & Bondas, T. (2014). Nursing students' perspectives of the cause of medication errors. *Nursing Education Today, 34*, 434–440. doi:10.1016/j.nedt.2013.04.015

Webster, T. L. (2018). Promotion of critical thinking in students: An examination of current educational practices. *Radiologic Sciences & Education, 23*(2), 23–31.

Wonder, A. H., & York, J. (2017). Using an academic and practice partnership to teach and promote EBP. *Worldviews on Evidence-Based Nursing, 14*(3), 249–251. doi:10.1111/wvn.12218

Young, D., & Seibenhener, S. (2018). Preferred teaching strategies for students in an associate of science nursing program. *Teaching & Learning in Nursing, 13*(1), 41–45. doi:10.1016/j.teln.2017.09.005

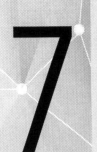

# Demonstrate Effective Interpersonal Communication and Collaborative Interprofessional Relationships

*WENDY H. HATCHELL*

> *We keep moving forward . . . opening new doors and doing new things.*
> —Walt Disney

## ▓ LEARNING OUTCOMES

At the end of this chapter, the learner will be able to

1. Describe the importance of establishing collaborative interpersonal relationships.
2. Describe the barriers that impede communication.
3. Demonstrate communication steps for students' learning.
4. Describe communication tools to promote patient safety and quality.
5. List the steps comprising conflict management.

## ▓ INTRODUCTION

Being an effective communicator in the healthcare arena is an essential component of the nurse's role and begins at the baccalaureate level (American Association of Colleges of Nursing [AACN], 2008). One must be able to express not only the needs of the patient, but also those of the organization and workplace. Being able to convey one's knowledge, expertise, and understanding extends to communicating effectively as a team member working with those from other disciplines as well as being able to engage in conflict management to resolve issues. In this section, information is presented on how to work as a team member in collaborative interprofessional relationships, how to communicate, and how to resolve conflict when a breakdown in communication occurs.

## ▦ VALUE COLLABORATION

The Robert Wood Johnson Foundation defines *collaborative practice* as the active participants of each discipline in patient care, where all disciplines are working together and fully engaging patients and those who support them, and leadership on the team adapts based on patient needs. Effective interprofessional collaboration enhances patient- and family-centered goals and values, provides mechanisms for continuous communication among caregivers, and optimizes participation in clinical decision-making within and across disciplines. It fosters respect for the disciplinary contributions of all professionals (Tomasik & Fleming, 2015, p. 1).

Collaboration is needed more than ever in today's healthcare arena. This is due to the complexity of healthcare coupled with fragmented patient care. When collaboration occurs, care is coordinated and congruent. Effective, quality patient care occurs as a result of collaboration.

Interprofessional collaboration is of such importance that the Institute of Medicine (IOM), now known as the National Academy of Medicine, stated in *The Future of Nursing: Leading Change, Advancing Health* that "nurses must become full partners, with physicians and other health professionals, in redesigning health care, . . . . must be accountable for their own contributions to delivering high-quality care while working collaboratively with leaders from other health professions" (Institute of Medicine, 2011, p. 99).

The American Nurses Association states in *Code of Ethics for Nurses With Interpretive Statements* that, "The nurse collaborates with other health professionals and the public to protect human rights, promote health diplomacy, and reduce health disparities" (American Nurses Association, 2015, p. 31).

- Collaboration consists of building trust and respect.
- Collaboration brings together each discipline's perspective and expertise, which further build on and strengthen learning about the strengths of each discipline.
- Collaboration reduces gaps in coverage or oversight and prevents loss of key patient information resulting from lack of communication.
- It promotes quality and safety.
- Collaboration facilitates the Institute for Healthcare Improvement's (IHI; n.d., para 1) Triple Aim:
  - ▦ Improve the patient experience of care (including quality and satisfaction).

▪ Improve the health of populations.

▪ Reduce the per capita cost of healthcare.

## CREATE OPPORTUNITIES FOR COLLABORATION

The clinical nurse educator has an important role in promoting collaboration and making student nurses comfortable with interprofessional collaboration through guidance, coaching, and role-modeling. Steps needed for collaborative practice are listed in Exhibit 7.1.

---

**Exhibit 7.1   Key Practices and Steps in Collaboration**

1. Assess the environment.
2. Create clarity.
3. Build trust.
4. Share power and influence.
5. Develop communication skills.
6. Engage in self-reflection.

Source: Robert Wood Johnson Foundation. (2008). *Turning point: Collaborating for a new century in public health* [Issue Brief]. Princeton, NJ: Author.

---

It is important to teach about collaborative practice. As a clinical nurse educator, allowing students to see collaborative practice actually being used is very effective. Students should practice speaking with professionals from other disciplines during the care of their patients. An excellent method used to prepare students is for them to read the progress/case notes and talk to other professionals about the patient while making rounds. An example would be discussing medication issues with the pharmacist when a patient is placed on nothing per os (NPO) status for an extended period of time due to a gastrointestinal issue.

## SUPPORT OPEN COMMUNICATION

*Communication* is the exchange of information, ideas, thoughts, behaviors, emotions, and perceptions from one person to another individual or group. Some thoughts on communication:

• It may be expressed in writing, electronically, by listening, speaking, or expressed through facial expressions and body language.

• One's communication may be perceived either positively or negatively, despite his or her intent.

• For communication to be effective, it should be received and interpreted as intended.

- To confirm that the correct message was sent and received, it is important to allow for and provide feedback opportunities. Feedback allows one to listen, reflect, explain, clarify, and summarize the message

## ▦ BE A ROLE MODEL

The clinical nurse educator must also be alert for any barriers that may impede the process of communication by blocking or distorting the intended message. These barriers may come from a person, the environment, or the organization (Borkowski, 2016).

Personal barriers may include the following:

1. Beliefs
2. Values
3. Prejudices/biases
4. Background: Socioeconomics, culture, prior experiences
5. Emotions
6. Perception
7. Inability to empathize (Borkowski, 2016)

   Environmental/organizational barriers may include the following:

1. Competition for time/attention
2. Multiple hierarchy levels
3. Philosophy
4. Complexity
5. Relationship status
6. Terminology (Borkowski, 2016)

## ▦ USE CLEAR COMMUNICATION

Effective communication is created and fostered in a climate of trust, respect, and empathy (Huber, 2018). This climate further creates and allows for clear, direct, and straightforward messages. Communication is an important tool to learn in nursing. A positive communication process fosters the organization's vision and goals; allows effective care coordination; provides quality and effective care; and promotes transparency.

| 7.1   Evidence-Based Clinical Teaching Practice |
| --- |
| A high percentage of medical errors are caused by lack of communication. A study conducted by Boston Children's Hospital found that 30% of preventable medical errors were reduced by implementing a communication/handoff tool (Starmer et al., 2014). |

| 7.1 Clinical Nurse Educator Teaching Tip |
| --- |
| As a clinical nurse educator, it is important to convey to students that they are communicating about themselves every day they are in the CLE. This includes behaviors such as care taken in appearance, response to patient needs, attentiveness, and motivation. |
| CLE, clinical learning environment. |

Tools have been developed to assist healthcare professionals to promote clear, positive communication. The following section discusses several different communication tools that students are taught in the clinical learning environment (CLE).

## SBAR (SITUATION, BACKGROUND, ASSESSMENT, AND RECOMMENDATION)

*SBAR* is a simple, effective communication tool that can be utilized and adapted to almost any patient care issue. Some key attributes of SBAR are the following:

- The use of SBAR is emphasized by The Joint Commission as the primary form of communication to use across disciplines, particularly for relying critical and pertinent information.

- The use of SBAR sets the communication standard to establish safe and quality patient care (Institute for Healthcare Improvement [IHI], 2011).

- When communicating with someone who is not physically with you, it is important to provide an "I" before SBAR: Identify oneself.

| 7.2 Clinical Nurse Educator Teaching Tip |
| --- |
| SBAR can be utilized in building concept maps or care maps to assist students to familiarize themselves with its use and formatting. |
| SBAR, situation, background, assessment, recommendation. |

SBAR teaches students how to group types of information, particularly patient information, into an organized format. This format structure simply places the type of information into easy, memorable, and identifiable categories. Use the SBAR format to notify a healthcare provider, particularly one who is not familiar with the patient, to provide a simple snapshot of necessary and pertinent information. An example is illustrated here:

- I—This is (name).

- S—I am taking care of . . . , a patient of . . . who was admitted with . . . This is the present situation.

- B—The patient has a past history of . . . .

- A—This is my assessment . . . .

- R—These are my recommendations; what are your thoughts . . . ?

| 7.3   Clinical Nurse Educator Teaching Tip |
| --- |
| Have students practice these techniques during simulation or in postconference to increase their confidence with it. |

## ▪ LISTEN TO LEARNER CONCERNS

*Debriefing* is another effective communication tool used throughout the curriculum to foster effective critical thinking in the classroom, skills laboratory, CLE, and during simulation. *Debriefing* is defined as

> a dialogue between two or more people; its goals are to discuss the actions and thought processes involved in a particular patient care situation, encourage reflection on those actions and thought processes, and incorporate improvement into future performance. The function of debriefing is to identify aspects of team performance that went well, and those that did not. The discussion then focuses on determining opportunities for improvement at the individual, team, and system level. (U.S. Department of Health and Human Services [HHS], Agency for Healthcare Research and Quality [AHRQ], Patient Safety Network [PSNET], 2018, para. 2)

Debriefing can be used effectively after simulation or any healthcare situation in the CLE. The clinical nurse educator understands that:

- As a learning tool, debriefing focuses on what went well and what did not to suggest appropriate changes needed for patient quality and safety.

- Debriefing begins by asking for each member's perspective. In some instances, patients are also involved in the process.

- The thoughts and actions behind the steps performed are analyzed.

- The main takeaway points and lessons learned influence future interventions (HHS, AHRQ, PSNET, 2018).

## ▪ DISPLAY SUPPORT

As healthcare has expanded, so has the need for *conflict resolution*. Unfortunately, even in the best CLEs, conflict is going to occur. Conflict generally has a negative connotation; however, when presented or viewed in a positive manner, it provides the opportunity to increase understanding and build trust and respect.

## ▓ MANAGE EMOTIONS

In today's healthcare environment, it is crucial to assist nursing students in developing conflict-management skills. When conflict is experienced, it affects relationships, the effectiveness of the organization, and the quality of clinical outcomes. Conflict must be addressed promptly. If conflict is not addressed promptly, it often leads to a decrease in staff morale, quality of patient care, teamwork, communication, and collaboration, as well as an increase in healthcare errors. This further leads to lack of trust and respect (Gerardi, 2015a). Exhibit 7.2 lists conflicts that need resolution.

---

**Exhibit 7.2  Conflicts Requiring Interventions**

- Substantive: main reason
- Procedural/structural: policy/decision hierarchy, step process
- Environmental context: organizational climate or organizational situation
- Relational: individual or group response to a situation (Gerardi, 2015c, p. 59)

---

## ▓ MANAGE CONFLICT

The first steps in handling and teaching conflict resolution involve obtaining knowledge:

- Self-awareness and management of emotions (emotional intelligence)
- Understanding of group and organizational dynamics
- Understanding of relational dynamic/models (Gerardi, 2015c)

  Further steps in conflict management involve the following:

- Watch for dysfunctional patterns.
- Create a safe place.
- Establish the purpose and direction of the meeting.
- Listen, listen, listen.
- When you or are the one initiating the conversation, use "I" statements.
- Ask questions.
- Acknowledge concerns and issues.
- Let the group or individual establish agreement/resolutions.
- Clarify what is possible and offer realistic solutions (Gerardi, 2015d).

| 7.2   Evidence-Based Clinical Teaching Practice |
| --- |
| Almost et al. (2016) found that transformational leadership and self-reflection of emotions and behaviors enable one to communicate a clear vision, inspire and motivate others, display respect, and reduce conflict. |

| 7.4   Clinical Nurse Educator Teaching Tip |
| --- |
| Role-modeling and role-playing conflict scenarios involving resolution are essential and assist students to learn professional behaviors. |

As a clinical nurse educator it is imperative to teach students about conflict and not to run away from it, but simply use it as opportunities for growth and self-reflection. Conflict resolution is a leadership skill needed by all educators.

## ▪ MAINTAIN AN APPROACHABLE DEMEANOR

Clinical nurse educators increase student satisfaction and learning when they are approachable. Being approachable means more than just being physically present to students. Approachability encompasses specific personal and teaching attributes that include:

- Be flexible in meeting individual student needs.
- Be prepared for the clinical learning experience.
- Be professional yet person centered.
- Be passionate about the role.
- Maintain a positive attitude (Matthew-Maich et al., 2015).

## ▪ RECOGNIZE LIMITATIONS

Clinical nurse educators take on the role because they want to be a part of forming the next generation of nurses. A study by Nguyen, Duke, and Forbes (2018) demonstrated that years of clinical practice were not related to role confidence. Janzen (2010) describes the role transition from clinician to educator as an introspective process that includes understanding oneself. This introspective process assists clinical nurse educators to identify with the role and live with a vision of role expectations. The role expectations include establishing an authentic therapeutic relationship with students by:

1. Demonstrating respect
2. Being genuine
3. Being there/being available

4. Accepting individuality

5. Having self-awareness

6. Maintaining boundaries

7. Demonstrating understanding and empathy

8. Providing support

9. Promoting equality (Gerardi, 2015b; Helming, 2013)

## ■ DEMONSTRATE EFFECTIVE INTERPROFESSIONAL COMMUNICATION

Effective interprofessional or team communication promotes quality patient care. Interprofessional communication is a practiced skill that includes specific elements of team building:

1. Establish goals.

2. Understand roles and responsibilities.

3. Use effective plans.

4. Engage in positive communication and interpersonal relationships.

5. Solve problems collaboratively.

6. Evaluate the outcome(s) (Cooper-Duffy & Eaker, 2017).

Another method used to demonstrate effective communication in the CLE with interprofessional colleagues is the interprofessional HUDDLE with students. *HUDDLE* stands for *h*ealthcare *u*tilizing *d*eliberate *d*iscussion *l*inking *e*vent.

HUDDLEs are used as a strategic planning moment most often at the beginning of a shift or at any time when needed to communicate plans, issues, and needs, as well as to conduct a problem analysis for the unit or team that day. During the HUDDLE, student participation can assist in understanding the nursing and interprofessional processes of patient care. Many times the SECURE communication method is used during the HUDDLE to communicate all necessary aspects of a situation. The SECURE acronym stands for:

S—Any security issues or safety issues?

E—Any supply equipment needs or issues?

C—Any patient or family, customer services, staffing needs, census?

U—Who is assigned what specific role if the unexpected happens?

R—Risk: Who needs to have a central line or catheter removed? Any falls?

E—Any unmet emotional needs, or for palliative or pastoral care (Dutka, 2016, p. 62)?

Many CLEs use interprofessional grand rounds. Grand rounds are usually performed by a group of interprofessional providers, who either walk from patient room to patient room or present patient cases in a conference area. The goal of grand rounds is for all disciplines to contribute to planning the most effective patient care for each case. Having student participate assists them in becoming comfortable in their role and with that of other healthcare professionals (Poore, Stephenson, Jerolimov, & Scott, 2017).

## ▦ COMMUNICATE PERFORMANCE EXPECTATIONS

Students need clear understanding of what is expected of them in the CLE and have experiences that are appropriate to their student learning outcomes (Vatanserver & Akabnsel, 2016). Expectations are communicated through the nursing program through syllabi, clinical checklists, and course and clinical nurse educator instruction. The student handbook should present a clear picture of the professional behavior expectations as well as violations that will warrant follow-up. Having students "prepared" for clinical learning experiences and providing guidance are key factors in meeting the students' learning outcomes and ensuring students' satisfaction with experiences (Helgesen, Gregersen, & Ostbye, 2016).

| 7.3   Evidence-Based Clinical Teaching Practice |
| --- |
| Anderson (2018) completed a grounded study with Australian RNs about precepting or teaching nursing students in the CLE. The study revealed that RNs perceive contributing to the professional development of students "a choice." |
| CLE, clinical learning environment |

## ▦ SUMMARY

Developing communication skills is crucial in a healthcare environment because of its impact on effective patient safety and quality care. Communication is the cornerstone of building therapeutic relationships with fellow colleagues and with patients. Communication extends into building skills in managing conflict and collaborative relationships. The chief components in communication are listening and building trust. Communication tools and skill acquisition further improve communication.

| 7.1   Case Study |
| --- |
| Upon assisting a student with electronic documentation of patient care, you overhear another student, who is on the computer and answering call lights, page the nursing assistant to get the patient in room 412 a bedpan. As the clinical nurse educator, what are the appropriate methods used to address this situation with this student and the other students in the clinical group? |

(continued)

---

**7.1  Case Study** (*continued*)

**Questions for Reflection:**

How does the nurse educator teach the difference between delegation and using a team approach?

How should the clinical nurse educator begin the discussion about the subject of prioritization in postconference?

---

## ▪ REVIEW QUESTIONS

1. The clinical nurse educator observes a student not coming forward with needed, pertinent information to a team member from another discipline. The clinical nurse educator should:

   A. Remove the student from the situation.

   B. Tell the student to talk with the team member privately.

   C. Assist the student in developing this skill.

   D. Discuss this situation with the student.

2. The clinical nurse educator observes and hears a nursing student say, "It is not my job to clean the soiled patient, it is the unlicensed assistive personnel's responsibility." The clinical nurse educator should:

   A. Discuss this situation in postconference.

   B. Find a private moment and a place to talk with the student one on one.

   C. Let this matter go for now because he or she is a good student.

   D. Discuss roles and responsibilities, teamwork, and resolutions with the group.

3. The clinical nurse educator is with a student administering medications through a comatose patient's nasogastric tube. The student is explaining everything to the patient. A medical resident is also present in the room and observes this. The medical resident asks: "Why are you talking to the patient, he is comatose?" The clinical nurse educator should:

   A. Speak with the medical resident's superior.

   B. Role-model the correct conflict response with the student present.

   C. Confront the medical resident without the student present.

   D. Pull the medical resident aside later and talk to her about the comment.

4. As the clinical nurse educator, several healthcare providers have come to you to say that the new group of nursing students is not providing appropriate and relevant information when queried by the nursing graduates. You have completed your assessment of the situation and determined that:

   A. A debriefing should be done with the students.

   B. Conflict resolution should be conducted between the staff and the healthcare providers.

    C. Educate/reeducate the students on utilizing SBAR (situation, background, assessment, and recommendation).

    D. Educate/reeducate the students on collaborative practice.

5. The performance assessment of a procedure you witnessed on one of your assigned nursing floors is being done by two of your students; the assessment is chaotic and has no direction. As the clinical nurse educator, you realize:

    A. You should provide additional procedural education and training.

    B. Establish debriefing to discuss what went well and what did not.

    C. Allow the students some time to collect themselves.

    D. Have the students to retake the fundamentals-of-nursing course.

6. The Joint Commission, American Nurses Association, and other organizations have determined this to be a core competency that begins at the baccalaureate level:

    A. Advocacy for the nursing profession

    B. Delegation and prioritization

    C. Performing quality-improvement projects

    D. Communication and collaboration

7. As you are making rounds on your assigned floor, you encounter several nursing students discussing a situation that occurred this week. You realize you need to implement conflict management. One of the most important skills you need to use is:

    A. Listening

    B. Building trust

    C. Understanding group dynamics

    D. Understanding educational dynamics

8. It is time for postconference and you notice that several of the students are not communicating with each other and you sense tension in the air. As the clinical nurse educator you should:

    A. Just let this past, they will work this out for themselves.

    B. Not become involved, pass this on to the course coordinator.

    C. Establish a conflict-management implementation.

    D. Manage your uncomfortable emotions.

9. An important concept and key component for nursing students to grasp and carry throughout their lifelong learning that is crucial in all aspects of communication is to develop:

    A. Leadership skills

    B. Communication skills

    C. Conflict-management skills

    D. Self-reflection skills

10. A student says: "I do not understand why you are making me go and talk to this person that I do not get along with in our clinical group, when you should be handling the situation." As the clinical nurse educator, you reply:

A. "What makes you feel that way?"

B. "You are the one accountable for your relationship."

C. "Remember, you need to develop your conflict-resolution skills."

D. "Avoidance is not going to make your problem go away."

## ▓ REFERENCES

Almost, J., Wolff, A. C., Stewart-Pyne, A., McCormick, L. G., Strachan, D., & D'Souza, C. (2016). Managing and mitigating conflict in healthcare teams: An integrative review. *Journal of Advanced Nursing, 72,* 1490–1505. doi:10.1111/jan.12903

American Association of Colleges of Nursing. (2008). *The essentials of baccalaureate education for professional nursing practice,* Washington, DC: Author. Retrieved from http://aacn.nche.edu

American Nurses Association. (2015). *The code of ethics for nurses with interpretive statements.* Silver Spring, MD: Nursebooks.

Anderson, C. (2018). Is provision of professional development by RNs to nursing students a choice? *Australian Journal of Advanced Nursing, 35*(4), 34–41.

Borkowski, N. (2016). *Organizational behavior, theory, and design in health care* (2nd ed.). Burlington, MA: Jones & Bartlett Learning.

Cooper-Duffy, K., & Eaker, K. (2017). Effective team practices: Interprofessional contributions to communication issues with a parent's perspective. *American Journal of Speech-Language Pathology, 26*(2), 181–192. doi:10.1044/2016_AJSLP-15–0069

Dutka, P. (2016). The huddle: It's not for football anymore. *Nephrology Nursing Journal, 43*(2), 161–162.

Gerardi, D. (2015a). Conflict engagement: Workplace dynamics. *American Journal of Nursing, 116*(4), 62–64. doi:10.1097/01.NAJ.0000463034.03378.e3

Gerardi, D. (2015b). Conflict engagement: A relational approach. *American Journal of Nursing, 115*(7), 56–60. doi:10.1097/01.NAJ.0000467281.59188.76

Gerardi, D. (2015c). Conflict engagement: A new model for nurses. *American Journal of Nursing, 115*(3), 56–61. doi:10.1097/01.NAJ.0000461823.48063.80

Gerardi, D. (2015d). Conflict engagement: Collaborative processes. *American Journal of Nursing, 115*(5), 66–69. doi:10.1097/01.NAJ.0000465043.48286.13

Helgesen, A. K., Gregersen, A. G., & Ostbye, R. A. K. (2016). Nurse students' experiences with clinical placement in outpatient unit—a qualitative study. *BMC Nursing, 15,* 1–6. doi:10.1186/s12912-016-0167-1

Helming, M. B. (2013). Relationships: Therapeutic relationships in holistic nursing. In B. M. Dossey, B. M. L. Keegan, C. C. Barrae, & M. B. Helming (Eds.), *Holistic nursing: A handbook for practice* (6th ed., pp. 439–462). Burlington, MA: Jones & Bartlett.

Huber, D. L. (2018). *Leadership and nursing care management* (6th ed.). St. Louis, MO: Elsevier.

Institute for Healthcare Improvement. (n.d.). *IHI triple aim initiative* [Policy brief]. Retrieved from http://www.ihi.org

Institute for Healthcare Improvement. (2011). *SBAR* [Policy brief]. Retrieved from http://www.ihi.org/resources/Pages/Tools/SBARTechniqueforCommunicationASituationalBriefingModel.aspx

Institute of Medicine. (2011). *The future of nursing: Leading change, advancing health.* Washington, DC: National Academies Press.

Janzen, K. J. (2010). Alice through the looking glass: The influence of self and student understanding on role actualization among novice clinical nurse educators. *Journal of Continuing Education in Nursing, 41*(11), 517–519. doi:10.3928/00220124-20100701-07

Matthew-Maich, N., Martin, L., Ackerman-Rainville, R., Hammond, C., Palma, A., Sheremet, D., & Stone, R. (2015). Student perceptions of effective nurse educators in clinical practice. *Nursing Standard, 29*(34), 45–52. doi:10.7748/ns.29.34.45.e9640

Nguyen, V. N. B., Duke, M., & Forbes, H. (2018). Nurse educator confidence in clinical teaching in Vietnam: A cross-sectional study. *Collegian, 25*(3), 335–340. doi:10.1016/j.colegn.2017.09.008

Poore, J. A., Stephenson, E., Jerolimov, D., & Scott, P. J. (2017). Development of an interprofessional teaching grand rounds. *Nurse Educator, 42*(4), 164–167. doi:10.1097/NNE.0000000000000351

Robert Wood Johnson Foundation. (2008). *Turning point: Collaborating for a new century in public health: An RWJF national program* [Issue Brief]. Retrieved from http://rwjf.org/en/libr

Starmer, A. J., Spector, N. D., Srivastava, R., West, D. C., Rosenbluth, G., Allen, A. D., . . . Christopher, C. P. (2014). Changes in medical errors after implementation of a handoff program. *New England Journal of Medicine, 314*, 1803–1812. doi:10.1056/NEJMsa1405556

Tomasik, J., & Fleming, C. (2015). *Lessons from the field: Promoting interprofessional practice* [White paper]. Princeton, NJ: Robert Wood Johnson Foundation. Retrieved from http://rwjf.org

U.S. Department of Health and Human Services, Agency for Healthcare Research and Quality, Patient Safety Network. (2018). *Debriefing for clinical learning* [Fact sheet]. Retrieved from http://psnet.ahrq.gov/primers/primer/36/debriefing-for-clinical-learning

Vatanserver, N., & Akabnsel, N. (2016). Intensive care unit experience of nursing students during their clinical placements: A qualitative study. *International Journal of Caring Sciences, 9*(3), 1040–1048.

# 8

# Apply Clinical Expertise in the Healthcare Environment

*BETTY ABRAHAM-SETTLES AND DEMICA N. WILLIAMS*

*An expert is someone who knows some of the worst mistakes that
can be made in his subject, and how to avoid them.*
—Werner Heisenberg

## ■ LEARNING OUTCOMES

At the end of this chapter, the learner will be able to

- Define *clinical expertise, preceptorship,* and *mentorship.*
- Differentiate between clinical expertise and clinical competence.
- Describe two strategic models used to assess clinical reasoning skills.
- Implement practices that organize the clinical day to optimize safe patient care and student learning needs.
- Identify strategies used to link theory to practice.
- Discuss a variety of ways to improve patient safety.

## ■ INTRODUCTION

Today's healthcare environment requires collaboration from an interprofessional team. Nurses are important members of that team. As a member of the interprofessional team, the nurse uses clinical expertise to promote positive healthcare outcomes. Clinical nurse educators are one of the most important influences in developing the next generation of nurses. Clinical nurse educators use clinical experiences, evidence-based practice (EBP), and patient preferences and values to teach and promote positive patient healthcare outcomes and student learning outcomes. There is some common terminology used by clinical nurse educators or nurses in healthcare organizations. Some of the terminology is clarified in Exhibit 8.1.

---

**Exhibit 8.1   Clinical Terminology**

*Precepting* is a common nursing education strategy. Responsibilities of the preceptor and preceptee are well defined by the educational and healthcare organizations. In some instances, contracts may be signed between the preceptor and school or healthcare facility. The clinical nurse educator's role is to outline specific learning outcomes for the student nurse to meet.

*Mentoring* involves an experienced nurse having a relationship with a less experienced nurse. Both parties must be willing to enter into a learning agreement. The relationship can be formal or informal and has the potential to last for years. The intent is for the inexperienced nurse to accomplish professional goals. When mentoring is successful, the goals may exceed those of the mentor (Grossman & Valiga 2017). When mentoring is successful, the protégé experiences many positive professional outcomes (Gordon, 2000).

*Clinical expertise means integrating a practitioner's accumulated knowledge from patient care experiences, formal education, and current evidence to make clinical decisions.* Clinical expertise refers to the clinician's cumulated experience, education, and clinical skills. Sackett, Straus, Richardson, Rosenberg, and Hayes (2002) assert that clinical expertise is part of the equation that explains EBP and research demonstrates that EBP leads to high quality of care and best outcomes (Jeffs, Beswick, Lo, Campbell, Ferris, & Sidani, 2013; Reigle et al., 2008).

Clinical expertise of clinical nurse educators is used to advantage when describing authentic clinical scenarios; a useful strategy that assists the students to develop their own clinical expertise (Hickman et al., 2014). Demonstrating the reality of the healthcare environment using authentic examples helps nursing students appreciate best practices. Integrating EBP into clinical examples for the students assists them to understand that the professional role always includes research. Nursing students begin to understand that evidence garnered through research makes a difference in clinical outcomes. Putting the pieces together using expertise, research, evidence, and patient preferences develops *clinical judgment.*

*Clinical judgment* develops over time. Nursing program applicants come with a wealth of general education, and nursing programs compete in attracting the most qualified students. However, in the clinical setting, didactic knowledge alone does not equate to competent nursing.

EBP, evidence-based practice.

---

Clinical expertise is developed over time using various tools. One such tool is *concept mapping*, which operationalizes a constructivist theory of learning (Gerdeman, Lux, & Jacko, 2013). In the clinical setting, concept maps are successfully used to assess content knowledge and students' thinking patterns. Studies demonstrate that concept mapping can develop students' *critical thinking* in preparation for meeting today's healthcare demands (Wittmann-Price, Reap Thompson, Sutton, & Eskew, 2013).

Nurses at all educational levels use EBP to improve patient care outcomes. To meet the demands of healthcare and further promote effective EBP utilization, the American Association of Colleges of Nursing (AACN) published a *Position Statement on the Practice Doctorate in Nursing (DNP)* with a recommendation. The recommendation hinged on the DNP degree becoming the terminal degree for nursing practice by

2015. According to Chism (2013), the National Organization of Nurse Practitioner Faculties (NONPF), the DNP degree is designed to prepare nurses to become proficient at the following (Marion et al., 2003):

- Evaluating EBPs for care
- Delivering care
- Developing healthcare policy
- Leading and managing clinical care and health systems
- Developing interdisciplinary standards
- Solving healthcare dilemmas
- Reducing disparities in healthcare

## ▪ MAINTAINING CURRENT PROFESSIONAL COMPETENCE

Clinical competence and expertise are not automatic rites of passage for nurses as they gain chronological yearly experience. Knowledge alone does not guide practice. To improve outcomes, knowledge needs to be translated into safe and appropriate clinical practice (Hickman et al., 2014).

To remain relevant to any area of practice, nurses need to practice and/or be lifelong learners in the clinical or specialty area in which they teach. Healthcare is constantly evolving related to newly discovered evidence and research findings. Therefore, clinical nurse educators must maintain their competence through continuous education beyond their initial basic nursing education (Miller, 2012). Certification in a specialty area is a means for clinical nurse educators to publicly validate their clinical knowledge (please refer to Chapter 1, CNE®cl Exam Specifics, for more information about certification).

Remaining active in the workforce is another opportunity for clinical nurse educators to validate and expand knowledge and to remain relevant in the classroom and clinical teaching arenas. Clinical nurse educators employed full- or part-time in a clinical or specialty area can keep abreast of changes in practice. Also, healthcare nurses are able to interact with clinical nurse educators and share their experiences. This broadens the knowledge of clinical nurses and helps them remain current in their practice.

## ▪ TRANSLATING THEORY INTO CLINICAL PRACTICE

Theorists such as Watson, Rogers, and Roy laid the foundation for nursing theory that is used by nurses today to guide care. Currentnursing.com defines *nursing theory* as:

> a set of concepts, definitions, relationships, and assumptions or propositions derived from nursing models or from other disciplines and projects a purposive, systematic view of

phenomena by designing specific inter-relationships among concepts for the purposes of describing, explaining, predicting, and/or prescribing. Additionally, *theory* can be defined as "a belief, policy, or procedure proposed or followed as the basis of action." Nursing theory is "an organized framework of concepts and purposes designed to guide the practice of nursing." The first nursing theories appeared in the late 1800s when a strong emphasis was placed on nursing education. Nursing theories are developed to explain and describe nursing care, guide nursing practice and provide a foundation for clinical decision-making. (2012, p. 1)

Theories provide nurses a framework to guide their thinking so the right questions can be asked to determine the best patient interventions. Nurses develop the skill of *critically deciding* the following:

• What to ask?

• What to observe?

• What to focus on?

• What to think about (Chism, 2013)?

Clinical nurse educators use theories in everyday clinical situations. When a clinical nurse educator explains patient discharge instructions with a student for a patient after an orthopedic procedure, what theory comes to mind? Roy's adaptation theory is applicable to use in discharge situations when a patient has to adapt due to mobility limitations. Highlighting the theory application for students assists them to better understand the essence of patient care.

---

**8.1   Evidence-Based Clinical Teaching Practice**

Rosinczuk, Koltvniuk, Gorska, and Uchmanowic (2015) prepared a case report demonstrating the usefulness of Sister Callista Roy's Model of Holistic Care. The report shows how nurses may use a nursing theory in the healthcare environment rendering everyday care for patients with MS. Clinical nurses are often unaware of the many times theories are applied to a plan of care. The model provides comprehensive provision of nursing services and does not limit contact with patients.

MS, multiple sclerosis.

---

Clinical nurse educators have the role of fostering theory-based inquiry in nursing students. Nursing students will enter an EBP workplace environment that links theory to practice.

## Using Best Evidence

EBP can lead to best practice and better outcomes. Melnyk and Fineout-Overholt (2015) identify the steps of the EBP process as:

• Cultivate a spirit of inquiry.

• Ask the burning clinical question in PICOT (population/patient, intervention/indicator, comparison/control, outcome, time frame) format.

- Search for and collect the most relevant best evidence.
- Critically appraise the evidence (i.e., rapid critical appraisal, evaluation, and synthesis).

Integrate the best evidence with one's clinical expertise and patient preferences and values in making a practice decision or change. To do this:

- Evaluate outcomes of the practice decision or change based on evidence.
- Disseminate the outcomes of the EBP decision or change.

Using the 6 A's as identified by Thompson (2017) in her blog may simplify the steps of EBP for students. Here are the 6 A steps:

- Assess.
- Ask.
- Acquire.
- Appraise.
- Apply.
- Audit.

Best practices are disseminated after the research process is complete. Dissemination does not determine whether the practice will be implemented. Barriers and cost of the implementation must be considered. Patient preferences and values also must be considered. Challenges to integrating best practice include the following:

- Organizational factors
- Characteristics of nurses
- The nature of the research (Polit & Beck, 2018)

## ▩ EFFECTIVE LEADERSHIP

Nursing students will be leaders in some capacity upon graduation. The leadership role may be as simple as being in charge of their group of patients or the charge nurse for a shift. Preparation for this role is a responsibility of the classroom and clinical nurse educators. Leadership is incorporated into the undergraduate curriculum; this is an indication of the importance of leadership skills for the graduate nurse. Some believe that nurses are born leaders. Florence Nightingale is referred to as a *born leader* (Knowler, 2011). The current realization is that a leader has to be developed (Scully, 2015).

Clinical nurse educators demonstrate leadership and how to be a change agent for nursing students. Nursing students have to be prepared to function in an ever-changing complex healthcare environment. It is important that clinical nurse educators understand and respond appropriately to practice issues in order to effect and lead change.

The most effective clinical nurse educators are those who can role-model effective handling of real-life experiences and promote positive change for the patients and the workplace. The mature, practicing clinical nurse educator has great potential as an educational leader (Adelman-Mullally et al., 2013).

Leadership development is a lifelong commitment for nurses and is a process that occurs throughout their careers (Grossman & Valiga, 2017). Nursing students and graduate nurses have to be given opportunities to serve as leaders. These opportunities may be provided in simulation experiences, scenarios, case studies, or clinical learning experiences (CLE). Leadership development requires skill development.

Providing nursing students with a variety of experiences to develop leadership skills is essential. Effective leadership empowers the student nurse to think outside of the norm. An example is to have the student nurse be the team leader of the day's clinical group. The student can demonstrate leadership skills when interacting with fellow students. The student is responsible for making the peer assignments and consideration must be given to peers' strengths, weaknesses, and course objectives. Leadership develops over time by doing, not just observing.

The clinical nurse educator assists in developing the next generation of nurse leaders. Grossman and Valiga (2017) identify characteristics that clinical nurse educators must possess to cultivate new leaders:

- Personal attention
- Role modeling
- Precepting
- Mentoring

## ▦ CLINICAL REASONING

Patient safety is reliant upon nurses' ability to "think on their feet." *Clinical reasoning* is developed during nursing education. Although the nursing language is ambiguous on definitions for *clinical reasoning* and *critical thinking*, they are necessary skills to have in today's healthcare environment. Being proactive versus reactive is a result of clinical reasoning skills. Strategies that promote the development of clinical reasoning skills include the following:

- Questioning
- Thinking aloud
- Feedback

Each nursing student's strengths and limitations guide the decisions of the clinical nurse educator. The clinical nurse educator in a healthcare facility develops nurses based on individual strengths. Opportunities are sought to challenge the student in performing according to set expectations of the job role.

| 8.1 Clinical Nurse Educator Teaching Tip |
|---|
| Meet each student where she or he is. Although your students may be at the same academic level, the range of their progress will differ. Some may meet expectations, whereas others may exceed expectations. In addition to the mandatory requirements, individualize each student's clinical objectives to empower students to pass the clinical portion of the class as well as the didactic portion. |

## ■ INTEGRATING BEST PRACTICE

In today's healthcare environment, it is not only necessary to render quality nursing care, but a nurse must demonstrate the economic benefit of the care (value-based care). Practice alone does not equate to economic value. This is evident with the clinical nurse specialist (CNS) role, which has been absorbed into a supervisory role because the current environment does not recognize the economic value of the position (Nickitas & Frederickson, 2015).

Formally, *knowledge translation (KT)* is defined by the Canadian Institutes of Health Research (CIHR; 2016, p. 1) as a dynamic and iterative process that includes the synthesis, dissemination, exchange, and ethically sound application of knowledge to improve health, provide more effective health services and products, and strengthen the healthcare system. The CIHR definition has been adapted by others and Polit and Beck (2018) further note that knowledge translation is a term associated with promoting best nursing practice at the bedside. Barriers to using EBP in knowledge translation include the climate of healthcare systems. More models of management mimic business models rather than the chief nurse model, which oversees the nursing portion of care in the business of healthcare. The emphasis on understanding research may not be a priority as much as the bottom line in healthcare environments.

The attitude of clinical practitioners has to be that the economic bottom line will be positive due to positive healthcare outcomes. Integrating best practices with clinical expertise, personal experience, and patient preferences will make EBP a more comprehensive concept than research utilization. Having a voice of inquiry is what will keep EBP a topic of discussion.

Clinical nurses have to ask relevant questions that address gaps or disparities in healthcare. Care must be rendered on the basis of best practice. Clinical nurse educators cannot solely rely on their expertise. As noted in Polit and Beck (2018), Sackett et al. (2002) defines *EBP* as "the integration of best research evidence with clinical expertise and patient values" (p. 1).

## ■ BALANCING PATIENT AND STUDENT NEEDS

Balance must also occur between patient safety and student learning needs. The clinical nurse educator continuously seeks ways to integrate safety while addressing the needs of the patient and the student. Many nursing schools incorporate Quality and Safety Education for Nurses (QSEN; 2018) competencies into their nursing curriculum. The QSEN competencies are listed in Exhibit 8.2.

---

**Exhibit 8.2  QSEN Competencies**

- Patient-centered care
- Collaboration
- Evidence-based practice
- Quality improvement
- Safety
- Informatics

QSEN, Quality and Safety Education for Nurses.

---

QSEN is just one specific way to develop a culture of safety that assists the student in becoming confident in the healthcare environment. Scenarios can be practiced in a simulation lab prior to going to the clinical area.

The Institute of Medicine (IOM; 2001) identified nine categories of opportunities to improve patient safety.

- User-friendly designs make it easy for nurses to follow directions and minimize errors.
  An example is equipment with additional accessories fitting into specific openings, which prevents user error (i.e., electrical surgical unit [ESU]).

- Use checklists and protocols to eliminate relying on memory.

- Take appropriate breaks to avoid relying on vigilance. Set alarms so that nurses can differentiate between an emergent alarm and nonemergent alarms.

- Practice teamwork and collaboration. Using documentation to facillitate the handoff procedure to another interdisciplinary team member is a good example. Teamwork and collaboration promote continuity of care.

- Safe practices should be instituted—such as wearing a red stole while administering medications to indicate that no one should communicate with the nurse during this time.

- Make the patient the center of his or her care. When the patient is an active participant in his or her own care, errors are less likely to occur.

- Anticipate the unexpected by using additional staff when warranted. An example is to schedule more staff than usual in an endoscopy suite when a new scope system is implemented and put in place. The additional staff can assist with any issues that may arise during a procedure.

- Design for recovery, which can be as simple as practicing for a disaster drill that involves the entire healthcare facility.

- Improve access to accurate and timely information. An example is having formulary information readily available during medication administration and any time throughout the workday. Clinical decisions will not be delayed with just-in-time information (Barnsteiner, 2011).

Introducing students to situations that may occur and how to respond to them has the potential to reduce errors. Organizations can assist in reducing errors by creating a "just culture." As Tocco and Blum (2013) note, the Just Culture Model for accountability is based on four questions:

- Was the clinician knowingly impaired?

- Did the clinician consciously engage in an unsafe act?

- Did the clinician make a mistake that three other clinicians with similar experience are likely to make under the same circumstances (substitution test)?

- Does the clinician have a history of committing unsafe acts?

Helping students recognize system vulnerabilities prepares them to work safely with patients. The trend is to move away from a punitive culture to a *just culture*. Here, the focus is placed on what went wrong and not who caused the problem (Barnsteiner, 2011).

---

| 8.2 | Clinical Nurse Educator Teaching Tip |
|---|---|

Life balance is also needed for clinical nurse educators; its relationship to nurse educators has been studied (Owens, 2017). According to Harris (1995) in Owens (2017), the nurse educator's perspective has an impact on how she or he views her or his own life balance. Current studies indicate moderate life balance overall, which contradicts the information on the nurse educator shortage published by the NLN (2013). Dissatisfaction may be directly related to the following:

- Workload

- Compensation

- Incivility experiences versus life balance issues (Owens, 2017)

*Burnout* is a real phenomenon for many nurses. The literature supports the existence of burnout in the nursing profession in general. Very little has been published addressing burnout in nurse educators (Shirey, 2006; Stamm, 2009). Life balance in today's healthcare environment may be based on an individual nurse's perceptions. Individual perception of life balance may determine whether a nurse educator admits to feeling burnout.

Nurse educators who set boundaries on their time may decrease the onset of feeling exhausted and overwhelmed. Time constraints are important for the nurse educator because of the multifaceted demands on their time associated with teaching, service, and scholarship. Additional stressors that affect nurse educators are heavy teaching workloads. Demographics may also affect the nurse educator's perception of life balance (Owens, 2017). Additional research is needed to address variables in life balance for nurse educators.

NLN, National League for Nursing.

## Using Technology

Nurses have to demonstrate competence in using technology when working in the healthcare environment. The Technology Informatics Guiding Education Reform (TIGER) initial mission was to create a vision and informatics agenda with the assistance of leaders from various nursing specialty organizations (Ball, Douglas, & Walker, 2011). Utilizing informatics continues to be a core competency for healthcare professionals in the 21st century.

Education reform at all levels allows nurses to become competent in technology. Williamson and Muckle (2018) note that most students have smartphones. Faculty understand that the healthcare environment has changed and will continue to do so in the future. Faculty are now users of various technological tools and designs. Technology is infused into the nursing curriculum at all levels. Strategies are developed and aimed at achieving competence in technology.

In preparing nurses to use informatics, the TIGER vision has two pillars:

- Allow informatics tools, principles, theories, and practices to be used by nurses to make healthcare safer, more effective, efficient, patient-centered, timely, and equitable.

- Interweave enabling technologies transparently into nursing practice and education, making information technology the stethoscope for the 21st century (Ball et al., 2011).

Nurses can use technology in the healthcare environment to review evidence and best practices.

Having access to computers in the workplace makes information readily available. An example is the use of SmartForms, which are designed to integrate nurses' clinical decision-making into their everyday tasks of assessing patients and documenting findings. Correctly designed systems can suggest actions at the time of documentation (Schnipper et al., 2008). Patient outcomes can be evaluated based on information technology infrastructures that integrate EBP into the workflow (Ball et al., 2011).

## ▩ SUMMARY

Clinical nurse educators use their expertise to assist nursing students to gain clinical competencies. Besides procedural skills, clinical nurse educators promote student competencies in theory application, EBP, technology proficiency, leadership skills, and safe clinical reasoning.

| 8.1 Case Study |
| --- |

The student is assigned to an 80-year-old female with a history of diabetes mellitus, hypertension, and hyperlipidemia. The patient reported fatigue in the past 3 days. The patient presents with a temperature that she has had for the last 24 hours and reports pain and burning with urination. The patient also reports frequency of urination. She is alert and oriented with no history of loss of memory or confusion. The patient is weak and unable to perform her ADL so she used her Life Alert button. When her son arrived at her apartment, she was confused. Personal/Social History: The patient lives independently in a retirement community. She is widowed and has a daughter and a son who are involved with her. Discuss the clinical questions you would ask the student to develop "nurse thinking." Have the student formulate and reflect before and after report, but before assessing the patient.

**Questions for Reflection:**

How will the clinical nurse educator begin the postconference group discussion about patient autonomy versus safety?

How can the clinical nurse educator role-model family inclusion without violating HIPAA? What patient safety measures should the clinical nurse educator discuss with the student?

ADL, activities of daily living; HIPAA, Health Insurance Portability and Accountability Act.

## ■ REVIEW QUESTIONS

1. The clinical nurse educator assesses the clinical decision-making skills of the student by which means?

   A. Care plan review

   B. Concept maps

   C. Debriefing

   D. Bedside questioning

2. Which of the following is considered in the integration of care in evidence-based practice (EBP)?

   A. Patient preference

   B. Family preference

   C. Expert opinion

   D. Physician expertise

3. What is the first step in the evidence-based practice (EBP) process?

   A. Ask the clinical question

   B. Spirit of Inquiry

   C. Collect the most relevant evidence

   D. Critically appraise the evidence

4. Which leadership characteristic of the clinical nurse educator involves demonstrating best practice?

   A. Mentoring

   B. Precepting

   C. Role modeling

   D. Personal attention

5. Which strategy helps develop clinical expertise?

   A. Use real-life scenarios

   B. Administer content tests

   C. Concept maps

   D. Review case studies

6. The doctor of nursing practice (DNP) degree trains nurses to become proficient in what area?

   A. Identify new procedures.

   B. Evaluate evidence-based practices for care.

   C. Research for breakthroughs.

   D. Develop interdisciplinary standards.

7. Which is the most effective tool for the clinical faculty member to use to teach concept mapping to a group of fundamentals-level nursing students?

   A. Review of exemplars from senior-level nursing students.

   B. Review of the clinical facility electronic health record (EHR) care plan.

   C. Review completed concept maps during postconference.

   D. Begin with teaching about creating a linear care plan.

8. Senior nursing students are asked to submit a topic for approval for an evidence-based practice project that they can implement on their clinical unit. Which student submission will be given back to the student for further clarification before proceeding with the project?

   A. Decreased use of indwelling Foley catheters decrease the incidence of catheter-associated urinary tract infections.

   B. Appropriately timed collection of stool samples from patients with suspected *Clostridium difficile* infection in order to correctly identify or rule out a hospital-acquired infection.

   C. The use of scheduled mouth care for mechanically ventilated patients decreases the incidence of ventilator-associated pneumonia.

   D. Biphasic defibrillators decrease the incidence of code blue situations in an acute care setting.

9. The clinical course coordinator is planning student–preceptor assignments for an upcoming semester by reviewing former student evaluations of nurse preceptors on a medical–surgical unit. When evaluating to determine whether or not preceptors would be asked to precept subsequent students, the clinical faculty finds which of the following is helpful in making concrete decisions about inviting preceptors to continue precepting students?

   A. The students make comments about relationships formed with the preceptor outside of work/school.

   B. The student's use of hospital policy and practice standards when performing new skills with the preceptor.

   C. The student's feedback on the complexity of patients being more than a student should care for while still studying.

   D. The student's opinion of how the unit is managed by the nurse manager.

10. With the shift to many clinical nurse specialists assuming supervisory roles in practice settings, which of the following job-related responsibilities is likely not to have been included in a traditional clinical nurse specialist academic program of study?

A. Role of change agent

B. Role of a leader

C. Role of manager

D. Role of clinical expert

## ▨ REFERENCES

Adelman-Mullally, T., Mulder, C. K., McCarter-Spalding, D. E., Hagler, D. A., Gaberson, K. B., Hanner, M. B., . . . Young, P. K. (2013). The clinical nurse educator as leader. *Nurse Education in Practice, 13*(1), 29–34. doi:10.1016/j.nepr.2012.07.006 N

Ball, M. J., Douglas, J. V., & Walker, P. H. (2011). *Nursing informatics: Where technology and caring meet.* London, EnglandLondon: Springer Verlag.

Barnsteiner, J. H. (2011). Teaching the culture of safety. *Online Journal of Issues in Nursing, 16*(3), 5. doi:10.3912/OJIN.Vol16No03

Canadian Institutes of Health Research. (2016). *Knowledge translation at CIHR.* Retrieved from http://www.cihr-irsc.gc.ca/e/29418.html

Chism, L.A. (2013). *The doctor of nursing practice: A guidebook for role development and professional issues.* Burlington, MA: Jones & Bartlett Learning.

Currentnursing.com. (2012). *Nursing theories: A companion to nursing theories and models.* Retrieved from http://currentnursing.com/nursing_theory/introduction.html

Gerdeman, J. L., Lux, K., & Jacko, J. (2013). Using concept mapping to build clinical judgement skills. *Nurse Education in Practice, 13*, 11–17. doi:10.1016/j.nepr.2012.05.009

Gordon, P. A. (2000). The road to success with a mentor. *Journal of Vascular Nursing, 18*(1), 30–33. doi:10.1016/S1062-0303(00)90059-1

Grossman, S. C., & Valiga, T. M. (2017). *The new leadership challenge.* Philadelphia, PA: F. A. Davis.

Harris, M. (1995). Assessing the quality of the working life of nurse educators in Finland: Perceptions of nurse educators and their spouses. *Journal of Advanced Nursing, 21*(2), 378–386. doi:10.1111/j.1365-2648.1995.tb02537.x

Hickman, L. D., Kelly, H., & Phillips, J. L. (2014). EVITEACH: A study exploring ways to optimise the uptake of evidence-based practice to undergraduate nurses. *Nurse Education in Practice, 14*, 598–604. doi:10.1016/j.nepr.2014.05.013

Institute of Medicine. (2001). *Crossing the quality chasm: A new health system for the 20th century.* Washington, DC: National Academies Press.

Jeffs, L., Beswick, S., Lo, J., Campbell, H., Ferris, E., & Sidani, S. (2013). Defining what evidence is, linking it to patient outcomes, and making it relevant to practice: Insight from clinical nurses. *Applied Nursing Research, 26*(3), 105–109. doi:10.1016/j.apnr.2013.03.002

Knowler, A. (2011). Florence had a vocation—She was born to lead. *Kai Tiaki New Zealand, 17*(4), 28–29.

Marion, L., Viens, D., O'Sullivan, A., Crabtree, M. K., Fontana, S., & Price, M. (2003). The practice doctorate in nursing: Future or fringe. *Topics in Advanced Practice Nursing eJournal, 3*(2), 1–8. Retrieved from http://www.medscape.com /viewarticle/453247_print

Melnyk, B. M., & Fineout-Overholt, E. (2015). *Evidence-based practice in nursing & healthcare. A guide to best practice* (3rd ed.) Philadelphia, PA: Lippincott Williams & Wilkins.

Miller, K. (2012). From the certified board nurse life care planning, licensure, specialty designation, certification, & accreditation. *Journal of Nurse Life Care Planning, 12*(4), 735–737.

Nickitas, D. M., & Frederickson, K. (2015). Nursing knowledge and theory: Where is the economic value? *Nursing Economics, 33*(4), 190–191.

Owens, J. (2017). Life balance in nurse educators: A mixed-methods study. *Nursing Education Perspectives, 38*(4), 182–188. doi:10.1097/01.NEP.0000000000000177

Polit, D. F., & Beck, C. T. (2018). *Essentials of nursing research: Appraising evidence for nursing practice* (9th ed.) Philadelphia, PA: Wolters Kluwer.

Quality and Safety Education for Nurses. (2018). *Competencies.* Retrieved from http://qsen.org/competencies/

Reigle, B. S., Stevens, K. R., Belcher, J. V., Huth, M. M., McGuire, E., Mals, D., & Volz, T. (2008). Evidence-based practice and the road to magnet status. *Journal of Nursing Administration, 38*(2), 97–102. doi:10.1097/01.NNA.0000310715.07850.68

Rosinczuk, J. K., Koltvniuk, A., Gorska, M., & Uchmanowic, Z. J. (2015). Application of Callista Roy Adaptation Model in the care of patients with multiple sclerosis-case management. *Journal of Neurological and Neuro Surgical Nursing, 4*(3), 121–129.

Sackett, D. L., Straus, S. E., Richardson, W. S., Rosenberg, W., & Hayes, R. B. (2002). *Evidence-based medicine: How to practice and teach EBM* (2nd ed.). Edinburgh, United Kingdom: Churchill Livingstone. Retrieved from https://nursingeducationexpert.com/what-does-clinical-expertise-mean-ebp

Schnipper, J., Linder, J., Palchuk, M. B., Einbinder, J. S., Postilnik, A., & Middleton, B. (2008). "Smart Forms" in an electronic medical record: Documentation-based clinical decision support to improve disease management. *Journal of the American Medical Informatics Association, 15*(4), 513–523. doi:10.1197/jamia.M2501

Scully, N. J. (2015). Leadership in nursing: The importance of recognizing inherent values and attributes to secure a positive future for the profession. *Collegian, 22*, 439–444. doi:10.1016/jcolegn.2014.09.004

Shirey, M. R. (2006). Stress and burnout in nursing faculty. *Nurse Educator, 31*(3), 95–97. doi:10.1097/00006223-200605000-00002

Stamm, B. H. (2009). *Professional quality of life: Compassion satisfaction and fatigue Version 5.* Retrieved from www.isu.edu/bhstamm

Thompson, C. J. (2017). Web blog post. *Use the 6A's to remember the evidence-based practice process.* Retrieved from http://nursingeducationexpert.com/evidence-based-practice-process

Tocco, S., & Blum, A. (2013). Just culture promotes a partnership for patient safety. *American Nurse Today, 8*(5). Retrieved from https://www.americannursetoday.com/just-culture-promotes-a-partnership-for-patient-safety

Williamson, K., & Muckle, J. (2018). Students' perception of technology use in nursing education. *Computer, Informatics, Nursing, 36*(2), 70–76. doi:10.1097/CIN.0000000000000396

Wittmann-Price, R. A., Reap Thompson, B., Sutton, S., & Eskew, S. (2013). *Nursing concept care maps for safe patient care.* Philadelphia, PA: F. A. Davis.

# Facilitate Learner Development and Socialization

TRACY P. GEORGE AND MARTY HUCKS

*Develop a passion for learning. If you do, you will never cease to grow.*
—Anthony J. D'Angelo

## ■ LEARNING OUTCOMES

At the end of this chapter, the learner will be able to

- Discuss ways to promote professional nursing behaviors and appropriate boundaries.
- Explain the importance of professional development and goal setting.
- Summarize techniques for stress management, self-care, and coping.
- Plan ways to incorporate quality-improvement processes.

## ■ INTRODUCTION

Since the creation of the first "training schools," nursing education has been steeped in clinical instruction. Most learners approach "clinicals" with some combination of excitement, joy, fear, and trepidation—realizing that this is where praxis will occur. In the clinical learning environment (CLE), learners perfect technical skills, apply knowledge, develop clinical judgment, try on leadership and advocacy roles, and solidify their understanding of humanity. In short, it is where they learn what it means to be a nurse. Our current understanding of socialization to the role of nursing demonstrates movement along the developmental continuum from basic survival mode to something resembling self-actualization and reflects the frequently painful transition from education to practice inherent in modern nursing. The importance of the clinical nurse educator and management of the CLE in the socialization and development of the neophyte cannot be stressed enough. This chapter examines a variety of topics related to the development of the professional nurse through the clinical arena.

## ▓ MENTORING LEARNERS

- The foundation of professional nursing practice includes the interplay of scope of practice, standards of practice, code of ethics, and specialty certification (American Nurses Association [ANA], 2015), which is experienced experientially by the student in the CLE.

- Mentoring learners in professionalism in the CLE involves an intentional relationship between the seasoned nurse/clinical instructor and protégé; it encourages lifelong learning among both parties and enriches the careers of each (Jakubik, Weese, Eliades, & Huth, 2017).

- The clinical nurse educator, within the context of the organizational setting, role-models and seeks out occasions for the learner to engage in and "try on" professionalism.

- Standards of practice (the nursing process) describe the broad expectations of any RN, regardless of setting; standards of professional performance delineate expectations of behavior in the role (ANA, 2015). Knowledge regarding standards of practice and professional performance is best transmitted through the CLE; missed opportunities occur when CLEs do not foster growth in learners' clinical reasoning capacity.

- Healthcare executives and nurse preceptors consistently report that new nurse graduates arrive to the healthcare arena lacking essential abilities in judgment and assessment (Jessee, 2016); students also recognize these deficiencies in themselves, which may contribute to high turnover rates within the first year of work.

- There is increased concern for ensuring ethical deportment in learners due to the complexity of the present healthcare milieu. Although knowledge regarding ethical codes is paramount in nursing education, current findings suggest a deficiency in exposure in most curricula (Numminen, Leino-Kilpi, van der Arend, & Katajisto, 2010). Simulation is beginning to be used as a tool for addressing ethical problems.

- Successfully teaching the *Code of Ethics* to learners and producing new nurses who are prepared for ethical decision-making involves integration of the material across the curriculum and formal training in the content for those who teach it (ANA, 2015).

| 9.1 Evidence-Based Clinical Teaching Practice |
| --- |
| Five phases of clinical teaching have been identified: beginning the role, strategies to survive in the role, turning point in the role, sustaining success in the role, and fulfillment in the role. Skilled nurse clinicians may find that they are initially ill prepared for supervising and evaluating students and may experience role strain. Strategies that help the transition include observing a clinical nurse educator at work prior to starting, having a mentor, assigning time for debriefing, and excellent communication with the course coordinator (Clark, 2013). |

## ▓ PROMOTING A LEARNING CLIMATE

- In a comprehensive review of the literature, Jessee (2016) found that learners repeatedly report that feeling accepted as part of the healthcare team is a crucial element in order for learning to occur in the CLE.

- The clinical learning climate may be conceptualized as a sociocultural environment consisting of physical, social, and cultural features and involving a power structure and human interactions that impact the ability of the unit to be a quality learning site (Jessee, 2016).

- Students may perceive unfair and disrespectful treatment from the clinical nurse educator, which may set the tone for a lack of respectful behavior in the CLE (Salminen, Rinne, Stolt, & Leino-Kilpi, 2017).

- In order to ensure a climate of inclusiveness, staff perceptions toward students and team-building opportunities must be considered in making determinations about using a potential site as a CLE (Jessee, 2016).

## ▓ PROMOTING PROFESSIONAL INTEGRITY

- For the 16th year, nurses have been ranked as one of the most honest and trusted professions in the United States (Brennan, 2017).

- Integrity is one of the values included in the ANA (2015) *Code of Ethics and Interpretive Statements*.

- The International Council of Nurses (ICN) *Code of Ethics for Nurses* states that an integral part of nursing is "respect for human rights, including cultural rights, the right to life and choice, to dignity and to be treated with respect" (ICN, 2012, p. 1).

- Academic dishonesty occurs in the clinical and classroom settings. In a study of 336 prelicensure nursing students, 64% had engaged in dishonest behavior in the classroom, and 54% had participated in dishonest behavior at least one time in the CLE (Krueger, 2014).

- In the CLE, a student may not report an error due to the concern about the repercussions of the mistake (Billings & Halstead, 2016). Students are often disciplined for medication errors (Disch, Barnsteiner, Connor, & Brogren, 2017). Barnsteiner and Disch (2017) urge nursing schools to move toward a fair and just culture, which requires students to be accountable for their actions but also encourages an investigation of system-wide issues that contribute to errors.

- Other examples of dishonesty in the CLE include the following:
  - ▨ A student in the CLE may submit a classmate's clinical assignment as his or her own work
  - ▨ Plagiarizing a source for a clinical assignment
  - ▨ Lying to a clinical nurse educator
  - ▨ Inappropriately documenting in the patient's record (Gaberson, Oermann, & Shellenbarger, 2015)

- When students engage in dishonest behaviors, there is the possibility that this behavior may continue in nursing practice (Palmer, Bultas, Davis, Schmuke, & Fender, 2016). In a survey of 1,296 nurses, Cohen and Shastay (2008) found that 37% of respondents did not report a medication error due to the concern that it may be harmful to them either personally or professionally.

- It is important for faculty to demonstrate integrity to students in the classroom and CLE (Eby et al., 2013).

---

**9.2  Evidence-Based Clinical Teaching Practice**

In a concept analysis of nursing integrity, the key components were honesty, ethical behavior, and professionalism. Devine and Chin (2018) identified the importance of faculty demonstrating integrity in their interactions with students.

---

## ▧ MAINTAIN PROFESSIONAL BOUNDARIES

- It is important for nurse educators to maintain appropriate relationships and boundaries with students. When nurse educators become friends with students outside the classroom, it may seem unfair to other students (Gaberson et al., 2015).

- Social media has become pervasive in society today. The ANA (2017) has developed guidelines for nurses using social media, which include the following:
  - ▨ Do not post identifiable patient information.
  - ▨ Maintain ethical nurse–patient boundaries.
  - ▨ Keep personal and professional social media accounts separate.
  - ▨ Be cognizant that employers may view social media postings.

- It is important to be aware of institutional policies regarding social media (Ashton, 2016).
- Ethical issues related to the use of social media:
  - ▪ Privacy and confidentiality
    - – Some nurses feel that they are protecting patient privacy if the patient's name is removed from social media posts, but this practice should be avoided. The nurse may provide the city and patient's age in the post, which could allow patient privacy to be compromised.
  - ▪ Nonmaleficence
    - – Posting information about a patient's condition could cause embarrassment to the patient. Remember that social media posts are permanent.
  - ▪ Professional integrity
    - – Befriending a patient on social media can compromise professional integrity.
    - – It is important for nurses to follow institutional policies regarding the use of social media (Henderson & Dahnke, 2015).
- When terminating the nurse–patient relationship, it may be tempting for nurses to connect with patients through social media, but this action violates professional boundaries (Ashton, 2016).
- Nurse educators should avoid being friends with students on personal social media sites. However, nurse educators may create professional social media accounts for use only with students in order to answer nursing questions in an interactive forum (Gaberson et al., 2015).

---

**9.1   Clinical Nurse Educator Teaching Tip**

It is important to role-model professional dress, behavior, and actions to students. Instead of giving out your cell phone number, encourage students to contact you via email or schedule meetings during office hours. Avoid friending students on social media or meeting students for meals or social outings. Students are watching your actions and how you delineate professional boundaries.

---

## ▪ ENCOURAGE ONGOING PROFESSIONAL DEVELOPMENT IN LEARNERS

- Nurse residencies and externships provide a formal way for nursing students and graduate nurses to improve the transition to practice as an RN. There is a need for all nurses to engage in lifelong learning (Gaberson & Langston, 2017).

- Technology is important in formal graduate educational programs, as well as for continuing education and lifelong learning. Technology can be used to "strengthen and support the teaching–learning experience, the transition from student to practitioner, and the shared investment with clinical practice in preparing lifelong learners with the knowledge, skills, and commitment to improve the system of care and its success in improving the health of the public" (Bellack & Thibault, 2016, p. 4).

- Career planning can encourage nurses to create goals for lifelong learning, and are used by organizations for succession planning (Webb, Diamond-Wells, & Jeffs, 2017).

---

**9.3  Evidence-Based Clinical Teaching Practice**

Journal clubs can be used to encourage professional development in nursing students. A series of five journal clubs over a 12-month period for second-degree prelicensure nursing students assisted in the socialization of students to nursing; they were found to be "valuable in cultivating clinical inquiry and lifelong learning" (Scherzer, Shaffer, Maceyko, & Webb, 2015, p. 226).

---

## ▪ ASSIST LEARNERS IN EFFECTIVE USE OF SELF-ASSESSMENT AND PROFESSIONAL GOAL-SETTING FOR ONGOING SELF-IMPROVEMENT

- Goal-setting, self-monitoring, self-regulation, and awareness of one's strengths and weaknesses are just some of the aspects of metacognition, a pattern of thinking that improves clinical decision-making (Kuiper, Murdock, & Grant, 2010). The use of feedback in relation to standards defines self-assessment and is crucial for professional growth (van der Leeuw & Slootweg, 2013).

- The literature shows inconsistencies in students' capacity to self-evaluate; Yeo, Steven, Pearson, and Price (2010) observed that even when nursing students felt proficient in a skill set, self-assessment was influenced by many factors, including modesty. However, as student-centered learning is desirable and self-assessment contributes to this as well as to professional development, it should be incorporated as part of reflective practice. The clinical nurse educator can facilitate the process by encouraging/giving the learner permission to be as accurate as possible.

- Truthful and fair negative feedback provided by the clinical nurse educator has been shown to increase learners' ability to correctly self-evaluate their performance, and even accurate positive feedback led to inflated self-assessment (Plakht, Shiyovich, Nusbaum, & Raizer, 2013).

- Self-evaluation is new to most students and involves a shift in roles. Providing a document that guides or prompts self-reflection as appropriate to the setting or course is useful (Siles-González &

Solano-Ruiz, 2016). For example, a checklist that incorporates questions such as "What was done well?" and "What needs improvement?" may facilitate student growth and insight.

## ▨ CREATE LEARNING ENVIRONMENTS THAT ARE FOCUSED ON SOCIALIZATION TO THE ROLE OF THE NURSE

- Many novice nurses report that their educational preparation was insufficient or incongruent with what is actually needed in the workforce. Some clinical environments push student learners toward assuming the role of nurses' aides in the CLE, thereby failing to foster socialization to the role of RN (Lovecchio, DiMattio, & Hudacek, 2015). "Reality shock" can set in when the new nurse discovers that his or her clinical skills are inadequate to the task.

- The CLE is frequently a stressful part of nursing school for students, as they must serve in two roles: learner and worker. Individualizing the level of supervision based on the needs of the learner is helpful in reducing anxiety and promoting growth toward socialization (Papastavrou, Dimitriadou, Tsangari, & Andreou, 2016).

- It is important for the clinical nurse educator to have a strong sense of task orientation, which includes properly organizing and allocating clinical assignments, using assignments that allow the student to engage in skills germane to nursing and that teach clinical reasoning while meeting course objectives; the availability of the clinical nurse educator is also an important aspect of this process. Task orientation can be a strong predictor of student satisfaction with the CLE (Lovecchio et al., 2015). Traits of the clinical nurse educator that support the desired socialization in the student learner include attending, empathy, reframing, and self-disclosure (Jakubik et al., 2017).

- Academic-practice partnerships may have advantages over the traditional clinical prototype in encouraging role socialization (Lovecchio et al., 2015).

## ▨ ASSISTING LEARNERS IN CONSTRUCTIVE PEER FEEDBACK

- Giving and receiving feedback is an important component of learning and may include reflection on both areas of strength and weakness. Comments should relate to a specific behavior, skill/competency, decision, or attitude and never involve a "personal attack." Feedback should be given when the learning or event occurs.

- The learner receiving the feedback should be encouraged to take time to allow the content to "sink in" and to separate any emotional component; it is helpful for the "receiver" to put himself in the place of the "giver" in order to recognize the context and acknowledge the work that went into preparing the feedback. Both "receiver" and "giver" should bear in mind that the purpose of feedback is performance improvement and that the "receiver" has the freedom to choose what to do with it (van der Leeuw & Slootweg, 2013).

- Student learners have been used successfully in peer assessments involving Objective Structured Clinical Assessment (OSCA)-simulated settings. Participants reported decreased stress in being evaluated by their peers, as opposed to the clinical nurse educator; learners in the evaluator role described better appreciation for the evaluation process and increased knowledge of the standards or criteria used for appraisal. Preparation of the learners is crucial and should involve material on professionalism, appropriate assertiveness skills, and time observing the application of constructive feedback. If possible, an assessment guide should be provided (Wikander & Bouchoucha, 2018).

## ▦ INSPIRING CREATIVITY

- The ideal way to inspire creativity in learners is to model it; however, many clinical nurse educators may not be "in tune" with their own creativity, and the current environment discourages divergence, focusing more on testing and conformity (Soh, 2016). Time and a lack of other resources are also constraints, as well as the notion that creativity does not have a place in the scientific process (Marquis & Henderson, 2015).

- Creativity is expressed in many ways—from producing a new product or idea to finding a new solution to a problem; it may not always be recognized. However, its value in a complex healthcare system is becoming more appreciated.

- Discussing examples of creative practices and allowing time for reflection increase confidence and creativity.

---

**9.4  Evidence-Based Clinical Teaching Practice**

The Creativity Fostering Teacher Behavior Index (CFTIndex) describes nine functions and corresponding behaviors that increase learners' creative expression. A few examples include encouraging independence in learning, allowing the full expression of students' views, probing to encourage thinking, having students evaluate themselves, and offering support when a learner is frustrated (Soh, 2017).

---

## ▦ ENCOURAGING TECHNIQUES FOR STRESS MANAGEMENT

- Reflective journaling can be an effective stress-reduction technique. Composing poetry may be another way for students to decrease compassion fatigue and stress (Jack & Illingworth, 2017; Thomas, 2015).

- Finding balance in life is important so that work is not all-consuming. Prioritization in one's work and personal life is important to relieving stress (Thomas, 2015).

- *Mindfulness* refers to an increased awareness of the present moment, which requires a person to slow down in a busy environment. Mindfulness is associated with improved resilience in nursing, and it can be accomplished through meditation, yoga, tai chi, reflection, or guided imagery (Calisi, 2017).

- Mindfulness may be associated with decreased stress levels. In a 1-month pilot study, 5-minute on-site mindfulness sessions prior to each nursing shift resulted in decreased stress levels from baseline to the end of the research study, and the effect was maintained for a month after the intervention (Gauthier, Meyer, Grefe, & Gold, 2015). Mindfulness-based stress reduction sessions with new nurses decreased stress levels postintervention and at 6 months (Wang et al., 2017).

- Smith (2014) found that mindfulness-based stress reduction was effective in improving nurses' ability to cope with stress, and it increased their ability to provide improved patient care. This technique is also effective in reducing stress among students. In a systematic review of eight studies, mindfulness-based stress reduction techniques were effective at reducing stress in graduate students (Stillwell, Vermeesch, & Scott, 2017).

---

**9.5    Evidence-Based Clinical Teaching Practice**

Benson's relaxation response (RR), which includes the use of diaphragmatic breathing and a repetitive mental focus, was used in a pilot study of 46 nurses over an 8-week period. Although nurses did not have lower anxiety, depression, well-being, and work-related stress levels when using RR, nurses were more confident in teaching patients about this technique at the end of the study ($p < .001$; Calisi, 2017).

---

## ▦ ACTING AS A ROLE MODEL

- The stressful work environment in nursing can lead to "burnout" or "compassion fatigue" (Murphy, 2014).

- According to the American Holistic Nurses Association (2013), self-care is a core value of holistic nursing.

- Self-care includes reflecting on one's health and wellness, in order to increase the awareness of the signs and symptoms of stress. It can be difficult for some nurses to balance providing compassionate care to patients and performing adequate self-care (Smit, 2017).

- Healthy habits include proper sleep, nutrition, exercise, and fostering mindfulness (Murphy, 2014).

- Remember that laughter and play can also decrease stress (Smit, 2017).

- Nurses also need to take the time for spirituality, which may include reading, prayer, meditation, and/ or time spent in nature (Smit, 2017).

## ▨ EMPOWERING LEARNERS

- Clinical nurse educators need to act as facilitators of learning and encourage active engagement of students. Students who are actively involved in the educational process are more likely to meet the student learning outcomes and be able to apply the information in the CLE (Billings & Halstead, 2016).
- Student engagement is based on the seven principles for undergraduate education developed by Chickering and Gamson (1987):
  - ▨ Encourage faculty–student contact.
  - ▨ Develop reciprocity and cooperation among students.
  - ▨ Encourage active learning.
  - ▨ Provide prompt feedback to students.
  - ▨ Emphasize time spent learning.
  - ▨ Communicate high expectations.
  - ▨ Respect diversity in talent and learning styles.
- According to Bloom's revised taxonomy, there are four types of knowledge: factual, conceptual, procedural, and metacognitive (Anderson & Krathwohl, 2001). Procedural knowledge includes skills, techniques, and methods used in nursing.
- There are several techniques for the active engagement of students in the area of procedural knowledge.
  - ▨ In the CLE, having students create algorithms may assist them to understand and apply difficult clinical concepts (Billings, 2016).
  - ▨ Demonstration is another strategy for actively engaging students in the CLE (Billings, 2016). Demonstration can be used with clinical skills, projects, or presentations.
  - ▨ Students may also be taught to use imagery and mindfulness, along with practicing psychomotor skills in the laboratory setting (Billings, 2016). One example of imagery uses relaxation techniques.

## ▨ ENGAGING LEARNERS TO APPLY BEST PRACTICES

- According to the Institute of Medicine (2003, p. 3), "All health professionals should be educated to deliver patient-centered care as members of an interdisciplinary team, emphasizing evidence-based practice, quality improvement approaches, and informatics."

- The Quality and Safety Education in Nursing (QSEN; 2018) competencies are as follows:
  - ▦ Patient-centered care
  - ▦ Teamwork and collaboration
  - ▦ Evidence-based practice
  - ▦ Quality improvement
  - ▦ Safety
  - ▦ Informatics
- Participation in quality-improvement projects is one way to teach nursing students about quality improvement. In one study, senior nursing students were introduced to the quality-improvement process through participation in quality-improvement projects in a geriatric setting (Dotson & Lewis, 2013).
- Partnerships between academia and clinical practice can assist in ntegrating QSEN competencies into clinical practice, and they can better prepare nurses for clinical nursing practice (Koffel, Burke, McGuinn, & Miltner, 2017). For example, at a Veterans Health Administration medical center, local nursing students have actively participated in rapid-cycle quality-improvement projects.
- Postclinical conferences can be used to integrate QSEN competencies, improve critical thinking skills, integrate theory and clinical practice, and encourage leadership skills (Mohn-Brown, 2017).
- It is important for nurses to be leaders in evidence-based change. One framework that has been developed is RN LEADER?
  - ▦ **L**ead with evidence.
  - ▦ **E**ngage nursing colleagues to participate.
  - ▦ **A**ct: Attend staff meetings and involve the chain of command.
  - ▦ **D**etermine the best, evidence-based solution.
  - ▦ **E**valuate outcomes.
  - ▦ **R**evise the plan of action (Porter & Strout, 2016).

## ▦ SUMMARY

The clinical nurse educator's role is multifaceted and crucial to the future of nursing. It is important for clinical nurse educators to promote professionalism with learners, including teaching ethics, integrity, and respect. Boundaries are important to maintain between faculty and students as well as between nurses and patients, this issue is magnified with the prevalence of social media. The clinical nurse educator should role-model professional development and goal-setting and encourage this with students. Learners need to be encouraged to recognize their strengths and weaknesses and seek our opportunities for professional growth. Nursing is a high-stress career, and stress management, self-care, and coping are skills that are important for the clinical nurse educator to demonstrate for learners. The quality-improvement process is used extensively in healthcare today, and nursing students need to be exposed to and involved in these activities so that they are better prepared for their role in healthcare. The clinical nurse educator must prepare students for their future roles as nurses in a rapidly changing healthcare environment that is patient centered, includes teamwork and collaboration, incorporates evidence-based practice, encourages quality-improvement efforts, is focused on patient safety, and is enriched with technology (QSEN, 2018).

---

**9.1  Case Study**

The course coordinator for the population-focused and healthcare policy class introduced learners to the impact of poverty and other social determinants of health outcomes through lecture, an online game, small-group work, and a relevant YouTube video. A short in-class exercise demonstrated the truth that a majority (but not all) of nurses and nursing students hail from a middle-class background and operate from this value system. Learners were attentive and engaged. To complement this learning unit, a clinical simulation exercise was carried out in conjunction with the school of education that involved role-playing a month in poverty. Senior BSN and school of education learners were placed in predetermined roles and over the course of an hour "lived out" four 15-minute "weeks" in poverty, took on the role of various community agency employees, or served as observers/note takers in order to provide feedback. As intended, the exercise was chaotic, the room was noisy, a sense of despondency developed, and participants quickly became tired and irritable. Most students were somewhat harried during the exercise, but seemed to appreciate the intended lessons. One student, however, became visibly distraught and ran into the bathroom crying at the end of "week 2." Her friend explained that the exercise was too painful, reminding her of a past that she would like to forget, yet unfairly highlighting some aspects of living in poverty.

**Questions for Reflection:**

- How should the clinical nurse educator handle this situation?
- Was a "climate of respect" breached for this student?
- How could the clinical nurse educator guide this student in self-assessment?
- Will this student have difficulty socializing to the role of nurse?
- What could the clinical nurse educator have done to avoid this problem and how should the assignment be changed going forward?

---

## ▪ REVIEW QUESTIONS

1. The student asks the clinical nurse educator to eat dinner with the clinical group at a restaurant. The clinical nurse educator should:

   A. Accept the invitation but only stay for 30 minutes.

   B. Decline with no explanation.

C. Tell the students that it is better that they go to dinner by themselves.

D. Suggest a restaurant with a band and bar.

2. The clinical nurse educator has received a social media "friend" request from a student. What should the clinical nurse educator tell the student?

A. I would love to connect with you on social media.

B. I must decline your request in order to maintain faculty–student boundaries.

C. I cannot be your "friend" on social media while you are in this course, but you can ask me in a later semester.

D. I only accept "friend" requests from students who have A's in the course.

3. A nursing student wears a hijab due to her Muslim religion. What does the clinical nurse educator tell her in the clinical learning environment?

A. You must remove your hijab while in clinical. It is not part of your nursing uniform.

B. You may wear your hijab, but only if you explain it to each patient.

C. You may wear your hijab in clinical. I know that it is an important part of your religion.

D. You need to quit wearing your hijab due to concerns about infection control.

4. The clinical nurse educator wants to encourage active learning in the postclinical conference. Which of the following would indicate that the clinical nurse educator needs additional instruction in active learning strategies?

A. Lecture the students about the most common diagnoses encountered in the clinical learning environment.

B. Have each student present information about his or her patient.

C. Assign students a presentation topic for postclinical conference.

D. Play an educational game that relates to the diagnoses in the clinical learning environment.

5. Which of the following would indicate that a nursing student needs additional instruction in self-care?

A. I get 3 hours of sleep each night.

B. I eat a healthy diet.

C. I exercise for 30 minutes three or four times per week.

D. I meditate each day.

6. The clinical nurse educator hears a nursing student talking about how stressful the nursing program is. Which statement by the clinical nurse educator is most appropriate?

A. Mindfulness-based stress reduction can help with stress relief.

B. You have to learn to live with the stress. It will only get worse once you are a nurse.

C. I use energy drinks to cope with stress.

D. I try to just do the tasks for each patient and try not to connect emotionally with patients.

7. A nursing student turns in a concept map that is similar to another student's concept map. What is the best response by the clinical nurse educator?

A. You worked with your classmate, and teamwork is important in nursing.

B. Your patients had the same diagnoses, so I understand why your concept maps look similar.

C. Plagiarism is not acceptable in the clinical learning environment.

D. The concept map is not graded. In the future, be sure to turn in your own work.

8. The clinical nurse educator is concerned that a student is exhibiting incivility when the student engages in which activity?

A. The student looks up the patient's medications on a smartphone application (app).

B. The student texts a friend about dinner plans.

C. The student asks the assigned nurse about the time of a scheduled procedure.

D. The student requests permission to observe the wound care nurse's evaluation of his patient.

9. Which of the following is the best way to encourage active learning about the quality-improvement process?

A. Give a quiz on quality improvement during postclinical conference.

B. Encourage student participation in quality-improvement projects in the clinical learning environment.

C. Lecture on quality improvement during postclinical conference.

D. Give students an article on the Quality and Safety Education in Nursing competencies.

10. A clinical nurse educator is providing an orientation to new nursing students at the beginning of the semester. The educator encourages students to join one of the nursing student organizations on campus. How will joining an organization assist students to be successful in the nursing program?

A. Encourages students to socialize to the role of the nursing student.

B. Teaches job-searching skills.

C. Reviews anatomy and physiology content.

D. Permits students to go on trips to conferences.

## ▦ REFERENCES

American Holistic Nurses Association. (2013). *Holistic nursing: Scope and standards of practice*. Silver Spring, MD: Author.

American Nurses Association. (2015). *Code of ethics for nurses with interpretive statements*, Silver Spring, MD: Author. Retrieved from http://www.nursingworld.org/MainMenuCategories/EthicsStandards/CodeofEthicsforNurses/Code-of-Ethics.pdf

American Nurses Association. (2017). *Social media*. Retrieved from https://www.nursingworld.org/social/

Anderson, L. W., & Krathwohl, D. R. (Eds.). (2001). *A taxonomy for learning, teaching, and assessing: A revision of Bloom's taxonomy of educational objectives*. New York, NY: Longman.

Ashton, K. S. (2016). Teaching nursing students about terminating professional relationships, boundaries, and social media. *Nurse Education Today, 37*, 170–172. doi:10.1016/j.nedt.2015.11.007

Barnsteiner, J., & Disch, J. (2017). Creating a fair and just culture in schools of nursing . . . Part 2 of a two-part series. *American Journal of Nursing, 117*(11), 42–48.

Bellack, J. P., & Thibault, G. E. (2016). Creating a continuously learning health system through technology: A call to action. *Journal of Nursing Education, 55*(1), 3–5. doi:10.3928/01484834-20151214-01

Billings, D. M., & Halstead, J. A. (2016). *Teaching in nursing: A guide for faculty* (5th ed.). St. Louis, MO: Elsevier.

Brennan, M. (2017). *Nurses keep healthy lead as most honest, ethical profession.* Retrieved from http://news.gallup.com/poll/224639/nurses-keep-healthy-lead-honest-ethical-sprofession.aspx?g_source=CATEGORY_SOCIAL_POLICY_ISSUES&g_medium=topic&g_campaign=tiles

Calisi, C. C. (2017). The effects of the relaxation response on nurses' level of anxiety, depression, well-being, work-related stress, and confidence to teach patients. *Journal of Holistic Nursing, 35*(4), 318–327. doi:10.1177/0898010117719207

Chickering, A. W., & Gamson, Z. F. (1987). Seven principles for good practice in undergraduate education. *AAHE Bulletin, 39*(7), 3–7.

Clark, C. L. (2013). A mixed-method study on the socialization process in clinical nursing faculty. *Nursing Education Perspectives, 34*(2), 106–110.

Cohen, H., & Shastay, A. D. (2008). Getting to the root of medication errors. *Nursing2008, 38*(12), 39–47.

Devine, C. A., & Chin, E. D. (2018). Integrity in nursing students: A concept analysis. *Nurse Education Today, 60*, 133–138. doi:10.1016/j.nedt.2017.10.005

Disch, J., Barnsteiner, J., Connor, S., & Brogren, F. (2017). Exploring how nursing schools handle student errors and near misses. *American Journal of Nursing, 117*(10), 24–42. doi:10.1097/01.NAJ.0000525849.35536.74

Dotson, B. J., & Lewis, L. (2013). Teaching the quality improvement process to nursing students. *Journal of Nursing Education, 52*(7), 398–401. doi:10.3928/0148483420130613-01

Eby, R., Hartley, P., Hodges, P., Hoffpauir, R., Newbanks, S., & Kelley, J. (2013). Moral integrity and moral courage: Can you teach it? *Journal of Nursing Education, 52*(4), 229–233. doi:10.3928/01484834-20130311-01

Gaberson, K. B., & Langston, N. F. (2017). Nursing as knowledge work: The imperative for lifelong learning. *AORN Journal, 106*(2), 96–98. doi:10.1016/j.aorn.2017.06.009

Gaberson, K. B.,Oermann, M., & Shellenbarger, T. (2015). *Clinical teaching strategies in nursing* (4th ed.). New York, NY: Springer Publishing Company.

Gauthier, T., Meyer, R. M., Grefe, D., & Gold, J. I. (2015). An on-the-job mindfulness-based intervention for pediatric ICU nurses: A pilot. *Journal of Pediatric Nursing, 30*(2), 402–409. doi:10.1016/j.pedn.2014.10.005

Henderson, M., & Dahnke, M. D. (2015). The ethical use of social media in nursing practice. *MEDSURG Nursing, 24*(1), 62–64.

Institute of Medicine. (2003). *Health professions education: A bridge to quality.* Washington, DC: National Academies Press.

International Council of Nurses. (2012). *The ICN code of ethics for nursing practice.* Retrieved from http://www.icn.ch/images/stories/documents/about/icncode_english.pdf

Jack, K., & Illingworth, S. (2017). 'Saying it without saying it': Using poetry as a way to talk about important issues in nursing practice. *Journal of Research in Nursing, 22*(6/7), 508–519. doi:10.1177/1744987117715293

Jakubik, L. D., Weese, M. M., Eliades, A. B., & Huth, J. (2017). Mentoring in the career continuum of a nurse: Clarifying purpose and timing. *Pediatric Nursing, 43*(3), 149–152.

Jessee, M.A. (2016). Influences of sociocultural factors within the clinical learning environment on students' perceptions of learning: An integrative review. *Journal of Professional Nursing, 32*(6), 463–486. doi:10.1016/j.profnurs.2016.03.006

Koffel, C., Burke, K. G., McGuinn, K., & Miltner, R. S. (2017). Integration of quality and safety education for nurses into practice: Academic-practice partnership's role. *Nurse Educator, 42*(Suppl. 5), S49–S52. doi:10.1097/NNE.0000000000000424

Krueger, L. (2014). Academic dishonesty among nursing students. *Journal of Nursing Education, 53*(2), 77–87. doi:10.3928/01484834-20140122-06

Kuiper, R., Murdock, N., & Grant, N. (2010). Thinking strategies of baccalaureate nursing students prompted by self-regulated learning strategies. *Journal of Nursing Education, 49*(8), 429–436. doi:10.3928/01484834-20100430-01

Lovecchio, C., DiMattio, M. J., & Hudacek, S. (2015). Predictors of undergraduate nursing student satisfaction with clinical learning environment: A secondary analysis. *Nursing Education Perspectives, 36*(4), 252–254. doi:10.5480/13-1266

Marquis, E., & Henderson, J. (2015). Teaching creativity across disciplines at Ontario universities. *Canadian Journal of Higher Education, 45*(1), 148–166.

Mohn-Brown, E. (2017). Implementing Quality and Safety Education for Nurses in postclinical conferences: Transforming the design of clinical nursing education. *Nurse Educator, 42*(Suppl. 5), S18–S21. doi:10.1097/NNE.0000000000000410

Murphy, B. (2014). Exploring holistic foundations and alleviating and understanding compassion fatigue. *American Holistic Nurses Association Beginnings, 34*(4), 6–9.

Numminen, O. H., Leino-Kilpi, H., van der Arend, A., & Katajisto, J. (2010). Nurse educators' teaching of codes of ethics. *Nurse Education Today, 30*, 124–131. doi:10.1016/j.nedt.2009.06.011

Palmer, J. L., Bultas, M., Davis, R. L., Schmuke, A. D., & Fender, J. B. (2016). Nursing examinations: Promotion of integrity and prevention of cheating. *Nurse Educator, 41*(4), 180–184. doi:10.1097/NNE.0000000000000238

Papastavrou, E., Dimitriadou, M., Tsangari, H., & Andreou, C. (2016). Nursing students' satisfaction of the clinical learning environment: A research study. *BMC Nursing, 15*(44), 1–10. doi:10.1186/s12912-016-0164-4

Plakht, Y., Shiyovich, A., Nusbaum, L., & Raizer, H. (2013). The association of positive and negative feedback with clinical performance, self-evaluation and practice contribution of nursing students. *Nurse Education Today, 33*, 1264–1268. doi:10.1016/j.nedt2012.07.017

Porter, J. S., & Strout, K. A. (2016). Developing a framework to help bedside nurses bring about change. *American Journal of Nursing, 116*(12), 61–65. doi:10.1097/01.NAJ.0000508674.23661.95

Quality and Safety Education in Nursing Institute. (2018). *Quality and safety education in nursing*. Retrieved from http://qsen.org/competencies/

Salminen, L., Rinne, J., Stolt, M., & Leino-Kilpi, H. (2017). Fairness and respect in nurse educators' work-nursing students' perceptions. *Nurse Education in Practice, 23*, 61–66. doi:10.1016/j.nepr.2017.02.008

Scherzer, R., Shaffer, K. M., Maceyko, K., & Webb, J. (2015). Journal club for prelicensure nursing students. *Nurse Educator, 40*(5), 224–226. doi:10.1097/NNE.0000000000000165

Siles-González, J., & Solano-Ruiz, C. (2016). Self-assessment, reflection on practice and critical thinking in nursing students. *Nurse Education Today, 45*, 132–137. doi:10.1016/j.nedt.2016.07.005

Smit, C. (2017). Making self-care a priority: Caring for the carer. *Whitireia Nursing & Health Journal*, (24), 29–35.

Smith, S. A. (2014). Mindfulness-based stress reduction: An intervention to enhance the effectiveness of nurses' coping with work-related stress. *International Journal of Nursing Knowledge, 25*(2), 119–130. doi:10.1111/2047-3095.12025

Soh, K. (2016). Fostering student creativity through teacher behaviors. *Thinking Skills and Creativity, 23*, 58–66. doi:10.1016/j.tsc.2016.11.002

Stillwell, S. B., Vermeesch, A. L., & Scott, J. G. (2017). Interventions to reduce perceived stress among graduate students: A systematic review with implications for evidence-based practice. *Worldviews on Evidence-Based Nursing, 14*(6), 507–513. doi:10.1111/wvn.12250

Thomas, S. (2015). Stress reduction tips for nursing students. *Alaska Nurse, 66*(4), 12–13.

van der Leeuw, R. M., & Slootweg, I. A. (2013). Twelve tips for making the best use of feedback. *Medical Teacher, 35*, 348–351. doi:10.3109/0142159X.2013.769676

Wang, S., Wang, L., Shih, S., Chang, S., Fan, S., & Hu, W. (2017). The effects of mindfulness-based stress reduction on hospital nursing staff. *Applied Nursing Research, 38*, 124–128. doi:10.1016/j.apnr.2017.09.014

Webb, T., Diamond-Wells, T., & Jeffs, D. (2017). Career mapping for professional development and succession planning. *Journal for Nurses in Professional Development, 33*(1), 25–32. doi:10.1097/NND.0000000000000317

Wikander, L., & Bouchoucha, S. L. (2018). Facilitating peer based learning through summative assessment—An adaptation of the objective structured clinical assessment tool for the blended learning environment. *Nurse Education in Practice, 28*, 40–45. doi:10.1016/j.nepr.2017.09.011

Yeo, J., Steven, A., Pearson, P., & Price, C. (2010). Influences on self-evaluation during a clinical skills programme for nurses. *Advances in Health Science Education, 15*, 195–217. doi:10.1007/s10459-009-9192-0

# 10 Implement Effective Clinical Assessment and Evaluation Strategies

*RUTH A. WITTMANN-PRICE*

*Quality means doing it right even when no one is looking.*
—Henry Ford

## ■ LEARNING OUTCOMES

At the end of this chapter, the learner will be able to

- Demonstrate the use of appropriate assessment tools to determine achievement of learning outcomes.
- Differentiate the use of formative and summative evaluative processes.
- Select appropriate documentation strategies to record achievement of learning outcomes.
- Appraise the effectiveness of the clinical learning environment.
- Provide constructive student feedback to improve clinical decision-making.

## ■ INTRODUCTION

In many ways, assessment and evaluation in the clinical learning environment (CLE) are more complex than evaluation methods in the classroom because it is more difficult to judge behaviors than to test objectives. Effective assessment and evaluation in the CLE require different methods and faculty skill sets. To begin, the clinical nurse educator should review the general definitions of *assessment* and *evaluation* to better provide student guidance.

- *Assessment* is a process in which information is gathered to determine whether learning has occurred. Multiple methods may be used to gather this information, analyze the information, and interpret the findings (Fliszar, 2017).

- *Evaluation* is a systematic and continuous process in which information is gathered to determine the worth and value of the program, outcomes, and achievement of the learner (Fliszar, 2017).

- *Formative evaluation* is done at some point during an educational process and focuses on what has been completed and what can be improved (Crabtree & Scott, 2016).

- *Summative evaluation* includes observing or assessing students over a period and arriving at a conclusion about performance and assigning a final rating or grade (Oremann & Gaberson, 2016).

- *Standards* and *guidelines* are "statements of expectations and aspirations providing a foundation for professional nursing behaviors of graduates of baccalaureate, master's, and professional doctoral and postgraduate APRN certificate program. Standards are developed by a consensus of professional nursing communities who have a vested interest in the education and practice of nurses" (Commission on Collegiate Nursing Education [CCNE] Accreditation Manual, 2013, p. 23). Accreditation Commission for Education in Nursing (ACEN) defines *standards* as "agreed-upon rules to measure quantity, extent, value, and quality" (ACEN, 2018, p. 10).

- *Criteria* are "statements that identify the variables that need to be examined in evaluation of a standard" (ACEN, 2018, p. 10).

- *Competencies* are defined by the American Nurses Association (ANA; 2013) as "an expected level of performance that integrates knowledge, skills, abilities, and judgement" (p. 3).

- *Clinical competency* evaluation is a crucial element of practice professions with a clinical skills component (G. Harrison, 2015). Many times, in nursing education, clinical competency is based on Benner's (1982) novice-to-expert framework (Kelly et al., 2016).

Accurately evaluating a student nurse's competence is important because it ultimately reflects the capabilities of the graduate nurse and how easily she or he transitions into practice. Evaluation is part of the quality assurance of the nursing education received (Kajander-Unkuri, 2015). The American Academy of Colleges of Nursing (AACN; 2008) emphasizes the importance of prelicensure clinical nursing education:

The roles of the baccalaureate generalist include provider of care, designer/manager/ coordinator of care, and member of a profession. Nursing generalist practice includes both direct and indirect care for patients, which includes individuals, families, groups, communities, and populations. Nursing practice is built on nursing knowledge, theory, and research. In addition, nursing practice derives knowledge from a wide array of other fields and professions, adapting and applying this knowledge as appropriate to professional practice (AACN, 2008).

The CLE, which also includes the skill and simulation laboratories, is the place where the application of professional knowledge is evaluated and assessed to ensure appropriateness with professional nursing competencies.

Student learning in the CLE is most often assessed using evaluation tools that are criterion referenced as opposed to norm referenced. Table 10.1 demonstrates the difference in the two types of assessment processes.

| Table 10.1 Comparison of Criterion-Referenced and Norm-Referenced Evaluations | | | |
|---|---|---|---|
| | **Scoring** | **Focus** | **Results** |
| **Criterion-Referenced Evaluations** | Based on preset knowledge that students should master | Focused on specific learning domains | Reported in percentage of correct answers or achievements based on a preset standard |
| **Norm-Referenced Evaluations** | Based on ranking of students in a group | Focused on a broad range of learning tasks | Reported as percentile rank from high to low achievers in a group |

*Source:* Fliszar, R. (2017). Using assessment and evaluation strategies. In R. A. Wittmann-Price, M. Godshall, & L. Wilson (Eds.), *Certified nurse educator (CNE) review manual* (3rd ed., pp. 135–155). New York, NY: Springer Publishing Company.

Regulatory and professional nursing organizations set healthcare provider standards and criteria that are often used as the foundation of clinical assessments and evaluations. The Joint Commission and Det Norske Veritas are organizations that accredit healthcare organizations by verifying that standards are met. The Institute of Medicine (IOM; 1999) recommends that health professions use competency or outcome-based assessments. The outcomes recommended by the IOM include the following:

- Patient-centered care
- Informatics
- Evidence-based practice
- Interprofessional team approach
- Quality improvement (Greiner & Knebel, 2003)

The National League for Nursing (NLN) has published graduate nurse competencies, which fall into the following main themes:

- Human Flourishing
- Nursing Judgment
- Professional Identity
- Spirit of Inquiry (NLN, 2012)

The AACN also has nine outcomes or "essentials" for graduate nurses and these are the following:

1. Liberal Education
2. Leadership
3. Evidence-Based Practice
4. Information Management
5. Healthcare Policy, Finance, and Regulatory Environments
6. Interprofessional Communication and Collaboration
7. Clinical Prevention and Population Health
8. Professionalism
9. Baccalaureate Generalist Nursing Practice (AACN, 2008)

## ▦ USING A VARIETY OF STRATEGIES

Student learning outcomes (SLOs) in the CLE may be different, but are congruent with the associated course or classroom SLOs. Content learned in the didactic or classroom setting often "comes to light" in the CLE, but may be displayed in different ways. Because classroom learning many times is primarily to gain content, it can be effectively tested with assessments that lend themselves to cognitive knowledge acquisition. Objective testing and written papers are some of the main evaluation strategies used to assess classroom content achievement.

The CLE is a teaching–learning area where learning is accomplished, not only in the cognitive (knowledge) realm, but also in the psychomotor (skills) and affective (attitude) domains of learning. All three domains of learning may warrant different evaluation mechanisms. Student achievements in the CLE are often evaluated by faculty-made clinical evaluation rubrics, skills checklists, care plans or concept maps, through observation of clinical decision-making and professional behaviors, and consideration of interpersonal and interprofessional communication, simulation scenarios, and the Objective Structured Clinical Examination (OSCE; Traynor & Galanouli, 2015). The CLE is a wonderful milieu in which to assess the three domains of learning because they often culminate in clinical decision-making about patient care needs (Figure 10.1).

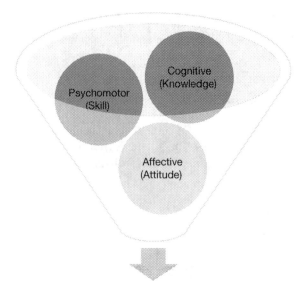

**Clinical Decisions About Patient Care**

**FIGURE 10.1** Clinical decision-making.

Currently, there is a movement to develop more standardized methods of clinical evaluation than have been used in the past. This movement has been prompted by several variables that include the following:

- Clinical nurse educators many times judge students on different standards (Oremann & Gaberson, 2016).

- Healthcare units are busy and clinical nurse educators are not always present to observe each student.

- Clinical nurse educators have different levels of preparation in student evaluation methods.

- Clinical nurse educators may be reluctant to clinically "fail" a student (Oermann, Kardong-Edgren, & Rizzolo, 2016).

Some types of commonly used clinical evaluation tools are listed in Table 10.2.

*Clinical Evaluation Rating Scales/Rubrics* can contain any number of specific items. Examples of general items that may be found on a clinical evaluation rating scale/rubric are the following:

- Responsibility and professionalism

- Planning and realization

- Assessment and diagnostics

- Systematic data collection from relevant sources

**Table 10.2 Commonly Used Clinical Evaluation Tools**

| Evaluation Tool | Most Commonly Used for | Rationale |
| --- | --- | --- |
| 1. Clinical Evaluation Rating Scales/ Rubrics | Often summative evaluations are composed of rating scales as opposed to checklists | Used to assess the students' end-of-course competencies, but can be used as formative evaluations; established on preestablished scoring criteria (Mertler, 2001) |
| 2. Clinical Skills (Competency) Checklists | Clarify and justify skill attainment | Lists skills required to be a competent nurse (Okupniak & Muller, 2017) |
| 3. OSCE | Provide a uniform basis for evaluation of students | "A method of clinical evaluation which is highly comprehensive, systematic and objective" (Vijayalakshmi & Revathi, 2017, p. 561) |
| 4. OSPE | OSPE integrates technical and theory "stations" to improve student clinical performance, prepare highly qualified and competent graduates, and increase decision-making abilities (Kaur, Thapar, & Kaur, 2017) | Used to evaluate clinical competence in all three domains: cognitive, psychomotor, and affective |
| 5. Observation | Recorded on clinical tools or anecdotal notes for formative and summative assessment | Watch and document students' behavior in all three realms of learning in the CLE (Hall, 2013) |
| 6. Care Plans | Learn the nursing process, nursing terminology, prioritization, and delegation | Used to assist students to follow a logical process to implement care (Patiraki, Katsaragakis, Dreliozi, & Prezerakos, 2017) |
| 7. Concept Maps | As an alternative to care plans, especially with upper level students | Allows the students to learn complex scenarios and use critical thinking skills by linking information (Bhusnurmath et al., 2017) |
| 8. Reflective Writing or Journaling | Lends itself to clinical learning experiences that are more in the affective domain | Assists students to self-reflect on how they feel about situations and what was learned (Mirlashari, Warnock, & Jahanbani, 2017) |

*(continued)*

| Table 10.2 Commonly Used Clinical Evaluation Tools *(continued)* | | |
|---|---|---|
| **Evaluation Tool** | **Most Commonly Used for** | **Rationale** |
| 9. Case Studies | Many times used for complex care or for clinical makeup when absences occur | Case studies can simulate, on paper, a clinical scenario for students; case studies can be presented as a singular case or unfold so that the complexity increases as students answer questions and make clinical decisions (Wittmann-Price, Thompson Reap, & Cornelius, 2017) |

CLE, clinical learning environment; OSCE, Objective Structured Clinical Examination; OSPE, Objective Structured Practical Examination.

- Prioritizing the patients' problems
- Appropriate technical skills in nursing interventions
- Discharge planning
- Performing appropriate, safe nursing interventions
- Disseminate appropriate education to individuals and families
- Assess the outcomes of patient education
- Communication skills with individuals, families, friends, and other health staff
- Inform nursing personnel about program and responsibilities
- Open to criticism
- Stress management and coping strategies
- Documentation of nursing care
- Using opportunities for learning and improving skills
- Responsibility and autonomy
- Knowing own strengths and weaknesses
- Teamwork and collaboration
- Inform the nurse personnel when student will leave the clinic
- Following the rules, ethical principles, and laws related to the care of individuals and families
- Respect for economic status, personal attitudes, and behaviors of individuals and families
- Respect for individuals' privacy during the process of nursing care (Gurkova, Ziakova, Zanovitova, Cibrikova, & Hudakova, 2018)

Nursing education programs may also choose to use the course SLOs as the items on the clinical evaluation rating scale/rubric to evaluate the student in the CLE. Clinical opportunities provide transfer of classroom knowledge to practice; therefore, both classroom and clinical performance need to be evaluated and many times clinical courses contain wording in the SLOs that include both learning environments. The evaluation of classroom and clinical performance is often done in tandem. There is much variation in clinical evaluation rating scales/rubrics and most are faculty made and reflect the culture of the educational organization. Many faculty-made clinical evaluation tools use a Likert-type scale. The Likert-type rating scale used for clinical evaluation can be simple as shown in Table 10.3.

| Table 10.3 Simple Rating Methods for Clinical Evaluations | | | | |
|---|---|---|---|---|
| 0 | 1 | 2 | 3 | 4 |
| Unsatisfactory | Sufficient | Good | Very Good | Excellent |
| Fail | Pass | Pass | Pass | Pass |

Source: Gurkova, E., Ziakova, K., Zanovitova, M., Cibrikova, S., & Hudakova, A. (2018). Assessment of nursing students' performance in clinical settings: Usefulness of rating scales for summative evaluation. *European Journal of Nurse Midwifery*, 9(1), 791–798. doi:10.15452/CEJNM.2018.09.0006.

Quantifying a clinical evaluation rating scale/rubric may decrease clinical nursing faculty subjectivity and provide students with a clearer picture of expectations. One of the most commonly used quantitatively enhanced scales/rubrics was developed by Bondy (1983). The scale/rubric has been used and modified many times since 1983 and includes descriptors, standards of procedures, quality of performance, and assistance (needed by the student from the clinical nurse educator). Table 10.4 shows the Bondy scale in its original form.

| Table 10.4 Bondy Scale | | | |
|---|---|---|---|
| Scale | Standard Procedure | Quality of Performance | Assistance |
| Independent | Safe Accurate<br><br>Effect ⎱<br>Affect ⎰ Each time | Proficient; coordinated; confident<br><br>Occasional expenditure of excess energy<br><br>Within an expedient time period | Without supporting cues |

*(continued)*

| Table 10.4 Bondy Scale (*continued*) | | | |
|---|---|---|---|
| **Scale** | **Standard Procedure** | **Quality of Performance** | **Assistance** |
| **Supervised** | Safe<br>Accurate<br><br>Effect ⎱ Each time<br>Affect ⎰ | Efficient; coordinated; confident<br><br>Some expenditure of excess energy<br><br>Within a reasonable time period | Occasional supportive cues |
| **Assisted** | Safe<br>Accurate<br><br>Effect ⎱ Most of the time<br>Affect ⎰ | Skillful in parts of behavior<br><br>Inefficiency and lack of coordination<br><br>Expends excess energy<br><br>Within a delayed time period | Frequent verbal and occasional physical directive cues in addition to supportive ones |
| **Marginal** | Safe but not alone<br>Performs at risk<br>Accurate—Not always<br><br>Effect ⎱ Occasionally<br>Affect ⎰ | Unskilled; inefficient<br><br>Considerable expenditure of excess energy<br><br>Prolonged time period | Continuous verbal and frequent physical cues |
| **Dependent** | Unsafe<br>Unable to demonstrate behavior | Unable to demonstrate procedure/behavior<br><br>Lacks confidence, coordination, efficiency | Continuous verbal and physical cues |
| **X** | Not observed | | |

*Source:* Bondy, K. N. (1983). Criterion-referenced definitions for rating scales in clinical evaluation. *Journal of Nursing Education, 22*(9), 376–382.

Rubrics are used as *criterion-referenced evaluations* and there are two types: analytic and holistic.

- An *analytic rubric* scores each criterion separately with time in between each item.
- A *holistic rubric* is scored in one process.

A template for a rubric is shown in Table 10.5.

Current clinical evaluation tools that have been developed and tested are described in Table 10.6.

Wu, Enskar, Lee, and Wang (2015) did a systematic review of the literature related to clinical evaluations (2000–2013) and found 14 studies.

**Table 10.5  Rubric Template**

|  | Beginning 1 | Developing 2 | Accomplished 3 | Exemplary 4 | Score |
|---|---|---|---|---|---|
| Criteria 1 | Description reflecting beginning level of performance | Description reflecting movement toward mastery level of performance | Description reflecting achievement of mastery level of performance | Description reflecting highest level of performance | |
| Criterion 2 | Description reflecting beginning level of performance | Description reflecting movement toward mastery level of performance | Description reflecting achievement of mastery level of performance | Description reflecting highest level of performance | |

Source: Mertler, L. (2001). Designing scoring rubrics for your classroom. *Practical Assessment, Research, and Evaluation, 7*(25), 1–8. Retrieved from http://pareonline.net/getvn.asp?v=7&n=25

**Table 10.6  Researched Clinical Evaluation Tools**

| Instrument | Year Developed | Researcher | Components | Results |
|---|---|---|---|---|
| SSPD | 2009 in Ireland | O'Connor, Fealy, Kelly, McGuinness, & Timmons, 2009 | Criterion referenced; generalizable; requires face-to-face teacher/learner meetings | Mixed-method study ($n = 29$ [students]; $n = 27$ [faculty]); positive perceptions, but takes time and faculty orientation |
| QLCCT | 2017 | Prion, Gilbert, Adamson, Kardong-Edgen, & Quint, 2017 | Measures 10 competencies on four levels of achievement | Good interrelater reliability and content validity |

QLCCT, Quint Leveled Clinical Competency Tool; SSPD, Shared Specialist Placement Document.

The study results were inconclusive as to reliability of clinical evaluation tools. Many tools used national organization standards as their foundation, but did not have effective statistical interpretation. Some of the main elements that are considered when evaluating nursing students include:

- Critical thinking skills
- Problem-solving
- Clinical decision-making (Patrick, 2019)

---

**10.1   Evidence-Based Clinical Teaching Practice**

When patients deteriorate, nurses need to know how to make acute clinical decisions. Liaw et al. (2018) developed and evaluated the psychometric properties of a CREST. The CREST measures clinical reasoning skills in recognizing and implementing nursing care during simulation for a patient who is deteriorating. The 10-item scale has a content validity of 0.93, an internal consistency of 0.92, Cronbach's alpha of 0.92, and an interrater reliability of 0.88. Most important, the usability of the tool was rated positively by the nurse educators.

CREST, Clinical Reasoning Evaluation Simulation Tool.

---

*Clinical skills (competency) checklists* are used to rate many psychomotor skills and nursing procedures. Evaluating nursing students' clinical "competency" is often difficult in the CLE due to its unpredictable and fast-paced environment. Nursing educational programs maintain checklists in both paper and electronic format and components of clinical skills (competency) checklists may include the following:

- Common skills deemed necessary for all RNs
- Critical skills or "must perform" requirements such as handwashing
- Procedural steps for a skill (Schuster, Stahl, Murray, Keleekai, & Glover, 2016)

---

**10.1   Clinical Nurse Educator Teaching Tip**

If electronic skills checklists are being used, (a) know the healthcare organizations' policy about cell phone use or (b) explain to the staff that if they see students using cell phones it may be legitimate use.

---

**10.2   Evidence-Based Clinical Teaching Practice**

Marvie, Maliheh, Tella, Smith, and Turunen (2017) studied how nursing students assess their own patient safety competence. The PaSNEQ was used to compare British ($n = 158$) and Finnish ($n = 195$) nursing students. Marvie and colleagues found that the majority of both British and Finnish students reported that their curriculum did not include a separate module for patient safety. All students ranked their competence to prevent patient safety incidents higher than they did their competence to act after errors were made. The study results suggest that clinical nurse educators should provide students with a more effective

*(continued)*

---

**10.2    Evidence-Based Clinical Teaching Practice (*continued*)**

practice environment that will prepare them with the patient safety skills needed to respond to work errors.

PaSNEQ, The Patient Safety in Nursing Education Questionnaire.

---

## Objective Structured Clinical Examination and Objective Structured Practical Examination

Objective Structured Clinical Examination (OSCE) and Objective Structured Practical Examination (OSPE) evaluation in the simulation laboratory can provide high-stakes type of testing. Although simulation methods are expanded upon as a clinical teaching tool in Chapter 4, Functioning Within the Education and Healthcare Environments: Operationalize the Curriculum, simulation as an evaluation tool is discussed here. OSCEs are becoming increasingly popular as an evaluation of clinical skill attainment. They can be done in a standardized method and recorded for review. Interrelater reliability is important to promote evaluation equity and consistency (Bagnasco et al., 2016).

---

**10.3    Evidence-Based Clinical Teaching Practice**

Hongli, Kamala, Tang, and Ng (2017) completed a cross-sectional study about nursing students' ($N = 85$) perceptions of OSCEs and found that nursing students felt OSCEs are reliable and valid methods to evaluate clinical competence. The majority of the participants thought the OSCEs were fair, organized, and covered competencies, although they did verbalize that OSCEs can be stressful. The researchers concluded that OSCEs provide constructive student feedback and improve competencies.

OSCEs, Objective Structured Clinical Examinations.

---

*Clinical observation* has long been used to evaluate student learning in the CLE. Clinical observation includes assessment of the student in all three learning domains. Both positive student observations and situations in which a student needs improvement need to be documented and shared via feedback. *Writing anecdotal notes* is a method of recording clinical behavior observed, but it is most likely done when negative behavior is observed that needs correcting (Hall, 2013). Anecdotal notes about students' observed behavior are often used as part of formative clinical feedback (Quance, 2016).

---

**10.4    Evidence-Based Clinical Teaching Practice**

Mackey et al. (2014) studied clinical observation by having senior nursing students act as standardized patients for other nursing students so as to gain insight and have the opportunity to use the clinical skills of observation, reflection, and evaluation to gain new insights into their own practice.

*Care plans* are used to evaluate the organization as well as the application of the nursing process and to guide nurses in the implementation of care (Yang, Wu, & Shan, 2018). Many times care plans are used with beginning nursing students to assist them in organizing their thoughts. Care plans are frequently written based on Gordon's functional health patterns to help students prioritize patient needs (Pieper et al., 2017). Care planning is based on North American Nursing Diagnosis Association (NANDA) nursing terms *nursing diagnoses* and *nursing outcomes* (Patiraki et al., 2017). Evaluation of care planning is important, especially for beginning students, to be able to demonstrate the proper use of the nursing process and the correct terminology (Wittmann-Price, Thompson, Sutton, & Eskew, 2013). Nursing care plans have been used for many years to evaluate the application of the nursing process and they can be an effective tool to promote positive patient outcomes (Khokhar et al., 2017). Using appropriate nursing diagnoses is also evaluated as part of care planning (Aydin & Akansel, 2013).

---

**10.5 Evidence-Based Clinical Teaching Practice**

Karadag, Caliskan, and Iseri (2016) investigated the effects of using case studies and simulated patients to teach students ($N = 70$) to plan nursing care. Data were collected by questionnaire and evaluating students' care plans and results demonstrated that the use of simulated patients assisted students to identify clinical needs and plan their nursing care.

---

*Concept mapping* has become commonplace and in many instances have replaced care plans. Concept maps assist the students to link together information in a nonlinear fashion. Evaluating concept maps requires one-to-one feedback (S. Harrison & Gibbons, 2013). Concept mapping also promotes creativity, problem-solving, and motivates students to learn (Chan, 2017).

*Reflective writing* evaluation is somewhat complex due to its subjective nature. Reflective writing, or journaling, lends itself to clinical learning experiences that are in the affective domain more than the psychomotor. Not only can reflective journaling assist students to better understand patient needs, but it can also decrease student anxiety (Mirlashari et al., 2017). Evaluating reflective writing or journaling is complex because it is usually subjective, and unless a rubric is developed to notify students that critical elements must be contained in their journal writing, the strength of this work is usually based on opinion. In addition, confidentiality needs to be addressed.

## Case Studies

Case studies are used as evaluative mechanisms for clinical knowledge attainment as part of the regular clinical requirement or as an absentee makeup requirement. Case studies promote critical thinking (Jones, 2017) and can be presented as:

- A single case study
- Unfolding cases
- Group case studies

Many times case studies are evaluated by ensuring the student uses the correct assessments provided to develop a reasonable plan of care and implements the necessary care in a writing exercise. Case studies can be extremely helpful in the analysis of patient data and in developing priorities (Wittmann-Price et al., 2017).

## ▦ IMPLEMENTING FORMATIVE AND SUMMATIVE EVALUATION

Students should be informed of the following:

- Course and clinical expectations in the form of a rubric, rating scale, objectives, competency checklist, and so on
- How they are doing as they progress (formative evaluation)
- What their final grade is and why (summative evaluation)

Students should not be surprised at the end of a CLE (summative evaluation) by an unsuccessful grade. Students at risk for being unsuccessful in the clinical practicum should have a learning plan, scheduled remediation, advisement, or coaching (formative evaluation) in place. The plan for improvement provides the student with a chance to be successful, but expectations need to be clear and consistent.

### Engaging in Communication With Course Faculty

Clinical nurse educators are most often expert practitioners who come into the teaching realm with intentions of "making a difference." The transition from practitioner to teacher is not always smooth. Communicating with the course faculty assists the clinical nurse educator to think in terms of academia as opposed to thinking in purely practice terms (Janzen, 2010). This communication process assists clinical nurse educators to become expert in their teaching roles.

Open communication with course faculty is also necessary for fair evaluation of students. Because most clinical components of nursing courses are evaluated on a pass/fail basis there is much room for subjectivity, as opposed to didactic learning, which is evaluated with letter or number grades. The communication process between the course faculty and the clinical nurse educator must be ongoing in order to fairly evaluate students. Expectations need to be consistent among students, between practice and academia, and between course and clinical nurse educators.

Many schools of nursing have a clinical nurse educator orientation day to assist in the communication process. Some of the communication tools used to assist clinical nurse educators are the following:

- A copy of the course syllabus
- Preceptor or clinical nurse educator manual
- The textbook(s) being used in the classroom
- A phone app for evidence-based practice reference

The clinical nurse educator should be able to reach the course faculty when an issue arises to discuss any situations about students, staff, or grading.

## Maintaining Integrity in Evaluation

Maintaining integrity in assessment and evaluation is more difficult today than ever before due to technically enhanced learning environments. *Integrity* can be defined as adherence to a code, especially of moral or artistic values. Faculty, students, or staff in the CLE can compromise evaluation integrity. A systematic review of the literature completed by Stonecypher and Willson (2014) of 43 articles about faculty's efforts to increase integrity mainly focused on classroom assignments and evaluations. The results of the Stonecypher and Willson study suggest that clear policies need to be put in place. This advice can be applicable to both the classroom and the CLE as many clinical assignments are written assignments.

Also, there is evidence that clinical errors are underreported due to fear of retribution. The IOM (1999) report demonstrates that errors occur due to systemic problems, one of which is failure to report. A study completed by Disch, Barnsteiner, Connor, and Brogren (2017) demonstrated that schools of nursing ($N = 494$) are not educating students to respond appropriately to clinical errors and "near misses." In addition, researchers found that few nursing programs have a policy for reporting and following up on student clinical errors or near misses and "significant work is needed if the principles of a fair and just culture are to shape the response to nursing student errors and near misses" (p. 24). Clinical nurse educators uphold integrity by providing a safe and just culture and teaching nursing students the proper steps in reporting errors and near misses. Process improvement plans for students may increase integrity rather than punitive clinical warnings.

---

**10.6 Evidence-Based Clinical Teaching Practice**

Mitchell, Baer, Ambrose, Folger, and Palmer (2018) studied workplace cheating and found that organizations may actually promote cheating by demanding high performance, employees' self-interested motives, and need for self-protection. Self-protection is a consequence of proving performance and avoiding negative consequences. The researchers in this sociological study found anger and self-serving cognition may lead to cheating.

## Providing Feedback

Formative evaluation should be done on an ongoing basis so students understand the practice areas in which they need improvement. Much of the current clinical teaching–learner evidence available concentrates on specific student competencies. Competency-based clinical education encompasses both formative and summative evaluation processes. Formative evaluations that identify an area needing improvement warrant a remediation plan. A remediation plan can be completed in the CLE, skills, or simulation laboratories and can improve students' skills, judgment, and clinical decision-making (Okupniak & Muller, 2017).

Providing feedback to students in the CLE should be both positive as well as instructive. Debriefing students in the CLE allows for reflection on what they have done well and what activity or thought process can be improved upon. Feedback can be done effectively in groups or one on one (Bonnel, 2016).

| 10.2   Clinical Nurse Educator Teaching Tip |
|---|
| Place in your syllabus the amount of time acceptable for email return, such as "Students can expect faculty to answer emails within 24 hours, excluding weekends and holidays." This way, expectations are clear. |

## Using Data

Using aggregated and trended data for process improvement is not new to programs of nursing. Data from one group of clinical learners are valuable but data trended over time about the CLE or clinical nurse educator demonstrate areas that need attention offer stronger evidence. Some of the issues that may arise have to do with the culture of the CLE. Organizations that are dedicated to a culture of safety may be better CLEs for students. Organizations that accept and invite students to learn will be evaluated highly at the end of the semester or academic term (Murray, Sundin, & Cope, 2018).

## Demonstrating Skill

The best practices in the assessment and evaluation of clinical performance come from

- Having valid and reliable evaluation tools (Table 10.7)
- Experience in clinical teaching
- CLEs that are user friendly to students and thereby decrease anxiety

## Assessing Learner Achievement

Students should have a clear understanding of the clinical expectations and how they will be evaluated. Most courses provide information in

| Table 10.7 Reliability and Validity of Evaluation Tools | |
|---|---|
| Validity | Reliability |
| Content validity—How well does the tool measure the intended SLOs? Criterion validity—Does the tool accurately predict future performance? Construct validity—How well can test performance be explained related to psychological characteristics? | Are test scores consistent group after group? |

Source: Fliszar, R. (2017). Using assessment and evaluation strategies. In R. A. Wittmann-Price, M. Godshall, & L. Wilson (Eds.), Certified nurse educator (CNE) review manual (3rd ed., pp. 135–155). New York, NY: Springer Publishing Company.

a clinical orientation session and outline expectations on the course or clinical syllabus. The clinical component of nursing courses is usually graded as a separate element within the total course grade on a pass/fail basis. Students sometimes question this assessment strategy and you may have heard student questions such as the following:

• Why can't the clinical portion of the courses have a letter grade?

• I am good in clinical, why do I have to retake that portion if I fail the course?

Clinical nurse educators are aware that the clinical practicum and classroom work are taught in tandem and that assigning letter grades to a clinical component can be done but would be difficult due to the nature of the process and the opportunity for subjectivity. Explaining to students that clinical skills need to be mastered by all correctly and there is not a differentiation of better and best in procedures, such as sterile technique, usually illustrates the concept for them. In addition, if a student is unsuccessful in a course, then he or she needs to retake both components (classroom and clinical) because being away from the clinical area may not serve the student well from a knowledge-application perspective. Also, a systematic review of medical literature demonstrated that pass/fail grading decreased student anxiety and increased motivation (Wasson et al., 2017)

## Using Performance Standards

Clinical performance can be assessed by any of the tools mentioned previously if they are applied consistently and as objectively as possible. Weaknesses should be identified in the CLE as early as possible to increase the chances of successful remediation as well as for patient safety. Performance standards are implicit in the clinical evaluation tools if they are applied consistently and as objectively as possible.

| 10.7   Evidence-Based Clinical Teaching Practice |
| --- |
| A concern for all clinical nurse educators is students' ability to assess patient acuity. Dalton, Harrison, Malin, and Leavey (2018) qualitatively studied what factors are included in nurses' ($N = 10$) assessments of patients who are physically deteriorating during their hospital stay. Some of the factors identified during interviews were interprofessional relationships, intuition, and interpretation of the MEWS system. Nurses relied on the numerical escalation of the MEWS system to identify the deteriorating patient, instead of their own clinical judgment. This research demonstrates that relying on tools and procedures may overshadow intuition. <br><br> MEWS, Modified Early Warning Score. |

## Documenting Learner Performance

In many nursing programs, learner clinical performance is documented on a pass/fail basis. Formative evaluations should be done with the appropriate feedback to provide the learner with mutually agreed-upon goals and learning objectives. Many clinical evaluation forms allow both formative and summative evaluations. Formative evaluations can be completed any number of times as needed to assist the student to improve in an area. Another form of documentation is *anecdotal notes.* Anecdotal notes are used to record clinical behavior, but are most often used to point out negative behavior that needs correcting (Hall, 2013). Anecdotal notes about students' observed behavior are often used as part of formative clinical feedback (Quance, 2016). Anecdotal notes can also provide positive feedback to students and foster confidence. As stated in Chapter 5, Functioning Within the Education and Healthcare Environments: Abide by Legal Requirements, Ethical Guidelines, Agency Policies, and Guiding Framework, anecdotal notes should be completed every day to record student.

## Evaluating the Clinical Learning Environment

The quality of CLEs is determined by many factors, including patient type, clinical nurse educator attributes, student preparation, staff expectations, and culture of the healthcare organization. Many variables need to be evaluated for nursing faculty to make an informed decision about future usage of a CLE. Figure 10.2 demonstrates some of the complexity of a CLE.

Students' evaluation and expectations of clinical nurse educators are important. Students should have the opportunity to evaluate their clinical nurse educator and the CLE. The clinical nurse educator evaluations should be shared with the clinical nurse educator by the course faculty or the nurse administrator in accordance with the educational organization policy. The evaluation of the CLE by the students should

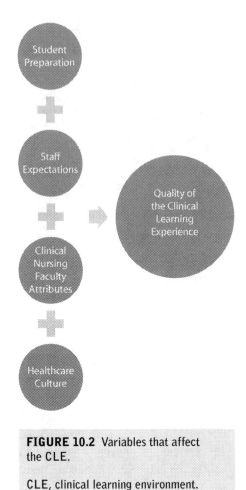

**FIGURE 10.2** Variables that affect the CLE.

CLE, clinical learning environment.

be shared in aggregate form with the healthcare organization director or unit director, but again this will depend on organizational policy. The clinical nurse educator should have a chance to evaluate the course faculty and the CLE in addition to evaluating each student. The course faculty should have the opportunity to evaluate the clinical nurse educator per organizational policy. The healthcare organization also should be included in the evaluation process to close the loop and either the director or staff can evaluate the clinical nurse educator and the students' effectiveness. This promotes an evaluation process that provides voice to all constituents. The data gleaned from the evaluations can be used to develop process-improvement strategies and enhance learning for the next group of students in that CLE. The evaluation process is depicted in Figure 10.3.

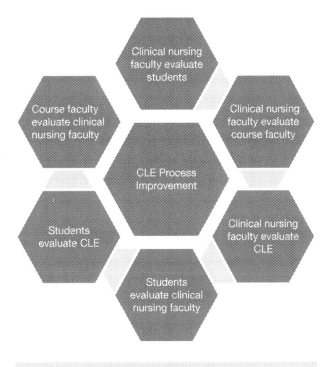

**FIGURE 10.3** The CLE evaluation process.

CLE, clinical learning environment.

---

**10.8   Evidence-Based Clinical Teaching Practice**

Lovric, Prlic, Milutinovic, Marjanac, and Zyanut (2017) studied nursing students' expectations of clinical nursing faculty and found in a 3-year longitudinal investigation that baccalaureate students (N = 34) expected their clinical nurse educators to be competent. *Competence* was defined as being knowledgeable in the following areas: teaching ability, clinical competencies, evaluation, relationships with students, patients, and healthcare team members, and personality traits.

---

Goldman and Mauk (2017) emphasize the importance of clinical nurse educator communication ability with staff and describe it succinctly as "the faculty person should communicate with the staff nurse who will be present with the student, what the student is expected to do and what the student's competencies are. The staff nurse should be comfortable with having the student perform the task" (p. 10).

---

**10.9   Evidence-Based Clinical Teaching Practice**

Jayalakshmi, Christian, Joshi, and Naidu (2017) studied the effects of mentorship on baccalaureate nursing students (N = 30). A quasi-experimental pre- and posttest of students' satisfaction was completed and found that students' self-confidence increased significantly with mentorship as did opportunities to demonstrate procedural knowledge. Students also

---

*(continued)*

| 10.9   Evidence-Based Clinical Teaching Practice (*continued*) |
| --- |
| reported that communication, empathetic treatment, individual attention, and overall clinical performance significantly increased. |

Unfortunately, today there are many schools of nursing that have little CLE choices due to the high volume of healthcare students. Establishing a positive relationship among the school, CLE, staff, faculty, and students is needed to evaluate clinical achievement without interference of negative environmental and structural variables.

## ▓ SUMMARY

Nursing clinical educational research is needed to establish new and innovative clinical assessments and evaluation tools. Over the years, nursing programs have effectively used clinical evaluation rating scales or rubrics, skills checklists, and case studies. OSCEs are becoming more popular as programs grow their simulation labs. Validity and reliability of rating instruments continue to be in the forefront of nursing research and assist in consistent evaluation processes. Clinical nurse educators serve the profession in a profound manner by being the "heroes of practice expertise" every day with students in a fast-paced complex environment. The insight clinical nurse educators provide academic education is invaluable and immensely assists the nursing education process to reach its goal of graduating competent and caring professionals.

| 10.1   Case Study |
| --- |
| A nurse educator is in the CLE with eight students in a beginning course. The students have had the fundamentals of nursing course and pharmacology course. One of the students draws up two different types of insulin incorrectly in one syringe. The clinical nurse educator questions the student prior to the student administering the medication and the student realizes the mistake. This "near miss" is fixed and the insulin is redrawn and administered correctly. |
| **Questions for Reflection:** |
| • What assessment and evaluative processes should occur to create a culture of safety? |
| • What should the clinical nurse educator report to the course instructor? |
| • How should the clinical nurse educator approach the near miss in group postconference to turn it into a learning experience? |

## ▓ REVIEW QUESTIONS

1. A clinical nurse educator is reviewing a student's care plans, concept maps, and anecdotal notes about the student to inform him of a grade. The clinical nurse educator is making a(n):

   A. Judgment

   B. Evaluation

C. Assessment

D. Remediation plan

2. The clinical nurse educator grades all the students' care maps in the clinical group and places them in a pile from best to worst and assigns grades. This a an evaluation process known as:

A. Assessment evaluation

B. Norm-based evaluation

C. Subjective evaluation

D. Criterion-based evaluation

3. Clinical nurse educators understand that the clinical evaluation process needs further research to develop better:

A. Validity

B. Reliability

C. Assessment skills

D. Criteria

4. The clinical nurse educator is developing a rubric for the students' care maps. The clinic nurse educator is placing a value for each component of the map on the rubric. The clinical nurse educator is making a(n):

A. Criterion

B. Evaluation

C. Assessment

D. Remediation plan

5. Regulatory and professional nursing organizations help establish:

A. Competencies and standards

B. Assessments for grading

C. Safe and unsafe behavior indicators

D. Pass/fail criteria

6. One of the advantages of evaluating clinical learning experiences compared to classroom processes is the ability to evaluate:

A. Cognitive learning

B. Psychomotor learning

C. Affective learning

D. Procedural learning

7. When using Objective Structured Clinical Examinations (OSCEs) for high-stakes evaluation, it is most important that the clinical nurse educator ensures:

A. The students are prepared.

B. The faculty understand the processes.

C. The conditions are standardized.

D. The standardized patients used display the symptoms.

8. The clinical nurse educator is using her anecdotal notes at midterm to debrief a student about an improvement process. The clinical nurse educator is developing a:

   A. Summative evaluation

   B. Formative evaluation

   C. Pass/fail decision

   D. Course grade

9. The clinical nurse educator is using the total assessment material at the end of the semester to assign a pass/fail grade to a student. The clinical nurse educator is developing a(n):

   A. Summative evaluation

   B. Formative evaluation

   C. Remediation plan

   D. Assessment

10. A clinical nurse educator is reviewing the standards for the clinical learning experience and finds them broad in scope. The clinical nurse educator should next review the:

    A. Student learning outcomes

    B. Criteria

    C. Course topical outline

    D. Syllabus

## ▦ REFERENCES

Accreditations Commission for Education in Nursing. (2018, March). *Accreditation manual.* Atlanta, GA: Author. Retrieved from http://www.acenursing.net/manuals/GeneralInformation_August2017.pdf

American Academy of Colleges of Nursing. (2008). *The essentials of baccalaureate nursing education for professional nursing practice.* Retrieved from http://www.aacnnursing.org/Portals/42/Publications/BaccEssentials08.pdf

American Nurses Association. (2013). *Competency model.* Silver Spring, MD: Author.

Aydin, N., & Akansel, N. (2013). Determination of accuracy of nursing diagnoses used by nursing students in their nursing care plans. *International Journal of Caring Sciences, 6*(2), 252–257.

Bagnasco, A., Tolotti, A., Pagnucci, N., Torre, G., Timmins, F., Aleo, G., . . . Sasso, L. (2016). How to maintain equity and objectivity in assessing the communication skills in a large group of student nurses during a long examination session, using the Objective Structured Clinical Examination (OSCE). *Nurse Education Today, 38,* 54–60. doi:org/10.1016/j.nedt.2015.11.034

Benner, P. (1982). From novice to expert. *American Journal of Nursing, 82*(3), 402–407.

Bhusnurmath, S. R., Bhusnurmath, B., Goyal, S., Hafeez, S., Abugroun, A., & Okpe, J. (2017). Concept map as an adjunct tool to teach pathology. *Indian Journal of Pathophysiology & Microbiology, 60*(2), 226–231. doi:10.4103/0377-4929.208410

Bondy, K. N. (1983). Criterion-referenced definitions for rating scales in clinical evaluation. *Journal of Nursing Education, 22*(9), 376–382.

Bonnel, W. (2016). Clinical performance evaluation. In D. M. Billings & J. A. Halstead, *Teaching in nursing: A guide for faculty* (5th ed., pp. 443–462). St. Louis, MO: Elsevier.

Chan, Z. C. Y. (2017). A qualitative study on using concept maps in problem-based learning. *Nursing Education in Practice, 24,* 70–76. doi:10.1016/j.nepr.2017.04.008

Commission on Collegiate Nursing Education. (2013). *Accreditation manual.* Washington, DC: Author.

Crabtree, J. L., & Scott, P. L. (2016). Peer Observation and Evaluation Tool (POET): A formative peer review supporting scholarly teaching. *Open Journal of Occupational Therapy, 4*(3), 1–17. doi:10.15453/2168-6408.1273

Dalton, M., Harrison, J., Malin, A., & Leavey, C. (2018). Factors that influence nurses' assessment of patient acuity and response to acute deterioration. *British Journal of Nursing, 27*(4), 212–218. doi:10.12968/bjon.2018.27.4.212

Disch, J., Barnsteiner, J., Connor, S., & Brogren, F. (2017). Exploring how nursing schools handle student errors and near misses. *American Journal of Nursing, 117*(10), 24–42.

Fliszar, R. (2017). Using assessment and evaluation strategies. In R. A. Wittmann-Price, M. Godshall, & L. Wilson, (Eds.), *Certified nurse educator (CNE) review manual* (3rd ed., pp. 135–155). New York, NY: Springer Publishing Company.

Goldman, M., & Mauk, T. (2017). The relationship between nursing students, program of nursing faculty and clinical facility nursing staff. *KBN Connection (Kentucky Board of Nursing Connection), 53*, 10–11.

Greiner, A. C., & Knebel, E. (2003). *Health professions education: A bridge to quality.* Washington, DC: National Academies Press.

Gurkova, E., Ziakova, K., Zanovitova, M., Cibrikova, S., & Hudakova, A. (2018). Assessment of nursing students' performance in clinical settings: Usefulness of rating scales for summative evaluation. *European Journal of Nurse Midwifery, 9*(1), 791–798. doi:10.15452/CEJNM.2018.09.0006

Hall, M. A. (2013). An expanded look at evaluating clinical performance: Faculty use of anecdotal notes in the U.S. and Canada. *Nurse Education in Practice, 13*(4), 271–276. doi:10.1016/j.nepr.2013.02.001

Harrison, G. (2015). Summative clinical competency assessment: A survey of ultrasound practitioners' views. *Ultrasound, 23*(1), 11–17. doi:10.1177/1742271X14550238

Harrison, S., & Gibbons, C. (2013). Nursing student perceptions of concept maps: From theory to practice. *Nursing Education Perspectives, 34*(6), 395–399. doi:10.5480/10-465

Hongli, S. G., Kamala, D. M., Tang, M. L., & Ng, K. C. E. (2017). Exploring nurses' perception towards objective structured clinical examination in Singapore: An exploratory cross-sectional study. *Singapore Nursing Journal, 44*(1), 8–15.

Institute of Medicine. (1999). Washington, DC: National Academies Press. Retrieved from http://www.nationalacademies.org/hmd/~/

Janzen, K. J. (2010). Alice through the looking glass: The influence of self and student understanding on role actualization among novice clinical nurse educators. *Journal of Continuing Education in Nursing, 41*(11), 517–523. doi:10.3928/00220124-20100701-07

Jayalakshmi, N., Christian, K., Joshi, S. G., & Naidu, S. (2017). Evaluation of the effect of clinical nurse mentors assigned to nursing students upon level of satisfaction regarding clinical teaching-learning process. *International Journal of Nursing Education, 9*(2), 40–45. doi:10.5958/0974-9357.2017.00033.2

Jones, T. (2017). Playing detective to enhance critical thinking. *Teaching and Learning in Nursing, 12*(1), 73–76. doi:10.1016/j.teln.2016.09.005

Kajander-Unkuri, S. (2015). *Nurse competence of graduating nursing students.* Academic dissertation. Turku, Finland: University of Turku.

Karadag, M., Caliskan, N., & Iseri, O. (2016). Effects of case studies and simulated patients on students' nursing care plan. *International Journal of Nursing Knowledge, 27*(2), 87–94. doi:10.1111/2047-3095.12080

Kaur, S., Thapar, K., & Kaur, N. (2017). Effectiveness of Structured Teaching Program (STP) on OSPE as a method in evaluation of clinical competency among nursing students. *International Journal of Nursing Education, 9*(2), 144–148. doi:10.5958/0974-9357.2017.00052.6

Kelly, J., Wilden, C., Chamney, M., Martin, G., Herman, K., & Russell, C. (2016). Improving cultural and clinical competency and safety of renal nurse education. *Renal Society of Australasia Journal, 12*(3), 106–112.

Khokhar, A., Lodhi, M. K., Yao, Y., Ansari, R., Keenan, G., & Wilkie, D. J. (2017). Framework for mining and analysis of standardized nursing care plan data. *Western Journal of Nursing Research, 39*(1), 20–41. doi:10.1177/0193945916672828

Liaw, S. Y., Rashasegaran, A., Wong, L. F., Deneen, C. C., Cooper, S., Levett-Jones, T., . . . Ignacio, J. (2018). Development and psychometric testing of a Clinical Reasoning Evaluation Simulation Tool (CREST) for assessing nursing students' abilities to recognize and respond to clinical deterioration. *Nurse Education Today, 62*, 74–79. doi:10.1016/j.nedt.2017.12.009

Lovric, R., Prlic, N., Milutinovic, D., Marjanac, I., & Zyanut, B. (2017). Changes in nursing students' expectations of nursing clinical faculties' competences: A longitudinal, mixed methods study. *Nurse Education Today, 59*, 38–44. doi:10.1016/j.nedt.2017.08.013

Mackey, S., Khoon, K. T., Ignacio, J., Pahlham, S., Mohamed, D., Rabiah, B., . . . Sok, Y. L. (2014). The learning experiences of senior student nurses who take on the role of standardised patient: A focus group study. *Nursing Education in Practice, 14*(6), 692–697. doi:10.1016/j.nepr.2014.10.003

Marvie, L., Maliheh, N., Tella, S., Smith, N., & Turunen, H. (2017). Self-assessment of patient safety competence: A questionnaire survey of final year British and Finnish pre-registration nursing students. *International Journal of Caring Sciences, 10*(3), 1212–1223.

Mertler, L. (2001). Designing scoring rubrics for your classroom. *Practical Assessment, Research, and Evaluation, 7*(25), 1–8. Retrieved from http://pareonline.net/getvn.asp?v=7&n=25

Mirlashari, J., Warnock, F., & Jahanbani, J. (2017). The experiences of undergraduate nursing students and self-reflective accounts of first clinical rotation in pediatric oncology. *Nursing Education in Practice, 25*, 22–28. doi:10.1016/j.nepr.2017.04.006

Mitchell, M. S., Baer, M. D., Ambrose, M. L., Folger, R., & Palmer, N. F. (2018). Cheating under pressure: A self-protection model of workplace cheating behavior. *Journal of Applied Psychology, 103*(1), 54–73. doi:10.1037/apl0000254

Murray, M., Sundin, D., & Cope, V. (2018). The nexus of nursing leadership and a culture of safer patient care. *Journal of Clinical Nursing, 27*(5/6), 1287–1293. doi:10.1111/jocn.13980

National League for Nursing. (2012). *Outcomes and competencies for graduates of practical/vocational, diploma, baccalaureate, master's practice doctorate, and research doctorate programs in nursing.* Washington, DC: Author.

O'Connor, T., Fealy, G. M., Kelly, M., McGuinness, A. M., & Timmons, F. (2009). An evaluation of a collaborative approach to the assessment of competence among nursing students in three universities in Ireland. *Nurse Education Today, 29*(5), 493–499. doi:10.1016/j.nedt.2008.11.014

Oermann, M. H., & Gaberson, K. B. (2016). *Evaluation and testing in nursing education* (5th ed.). New York, NY: Springer Publishing Company.

Oermann, M. H., Kardong-Edgen, S., & Rizzolo, M. A. (2016). Towards an evidence-based methodology for high-stakes evaluation of nursing students' clinical performance using simulation. *Teaching and Learning in Nursing, 11*, 133–137. doi:10.1016/j.teln.2016.04.001

Okupniak, C., & Muller, M. A. (2017). Facilitating learning in the clinical setting. In R. A. Wittmann-Price, M. Godshall, & L. Wilson, (Eds.), *Certified nurse educator (CNE) review manual* (3rd ed., pp. 135–155). New York, NY: Springer Publishing Company.

Patiraki, E., Katsaragakis, S., Dreliozi, A., & Prezerakos, P. (2017). Nursing care plans based on NANDA, nursing interventions classification, and nursing outcomes classification: The investigation of the effectiveness of an educational intervention in Greece. *International Journal of Nursing Knowledge, 28*(2), 88–93.

Patrick, A. M. (2019). Implement effective clinical assessment and evaluation strategies. In T. Shellenbarger (Ed.), *Clinical nurse educator competencies.* New York, NY: NLN.

Pieper, B., Monahan, J., Keves-Foster, M. K., Farner, J., Alhasanat, D., & Albdour, M. (2017). A quality improvement project: What first-year nursing students include in their nursing care plans for patients with acute or chronic wounds. *Ostomy Wound Management, 63*(19), 42–47. doi:10.25270/owm.2017.4247

Prion, S. K., Gilbert, E. G., Adamson, K. A., Kardong-Edgen, S., & Quint, S. (2017). Development and testing of the quint leveled clinical competency tool. *Clinical Simulation in Nursing, 13*(3), 106–115. doi:10.1016/J.ECNS.2016.10.008

Quance, M. A. (2016). Nursing students' perceptions of anecdotal notes as formative feedback. *International Journal of Nursing Education Scholarship, 13*(1), 1. doi:10.1515/ijnes-2015-0053

Schuster, C., Stahl, B., Murray, C., Keleekai, N. L., & Glover, K. (2016). Development and testing of a short peripheral intravenous catheter insertion skills checklist. *Journal of the Association for Vascular Access, 21*(4), 196–204. doi:10.1016/j.java.2016.08.003

Stonecypher, K., & Willson, P. (2014). Academic policies and practices to deter cheating in nursing education. *Nursing Education Perspectives, 35*(3), 167–179. doi:10.5480/12-1028.1

Traynor, M., & Galanouli, D. (2015). Have OSCEs come of age in nursing education? *British Journal of Nursing, 24*(7), 388–391. doi:10.12968/bjon.2015.24.7.388

Vijayalakshmi, K., & Revathi, S. (2017). Performance of nursing students in psychiatric nursing using Objective Structured Clinical Examination (OSCE) versus Traditional Practical Examination (TPE) - A comparative approach. *Asian Journal of Nursing Education & Research, 7*(4), 561–568. doi:10.5958/2349-2996.2017.00109.4

Wasson, L. T., Cusmano, A., Meli, L., Louh, I., Falzon, L., Hampsey, M., . . . Davidson, K. W. (2017). Association between learning environment interventions and medical student well-being: A systematic review. *JAMA, 316*(21), 2237–2252. doi:10.1001/jama.2016.17573

Wittmann-Price, R. A., Reap Thompson, B., & Cornelius, F. (Eds.) (2017). *NCLEX-RN® EXCEL: Test success through unfolding case study review* (2nd ed.). New York, NY: Springer Publishing Company.

Wittmann-Price, R. A., & Reap. Thompson B., Sutton, S. M., & Eskew S. R. (2013). *Nursing concept care maps for safe patient care.* Philadelphia, PA: F. A. Davis.

Wu, X. V., Enskar, K., Lee, C. C. S., & Wang, W. (2015). A systematic review of clinical assessment for undergraduate nursing students. *Nurse Education Today, 35*(2), 347–359. doi:10/1016/j.nedt.2014.11.016

Yang, H., Wu, M., & Shun, S. (2018). Care plan for resuming the physical activity of patients with pancreatic cancer and diabetes after surgery. *Journal of Nursing, 65*(1), 104–111.

# 11 Practice Test

1. A clinical nurse educator waits until the end of the academic term to evaluate the students on their clinical performance. She subscribes to a(n):

   A. Analytical rubric
   B. Totality assessment process
   C. Holistic rubric
   D. Formative process

2. When misconduct failures or dismissals are enacted, several steps must be taken by the clinical faculty to ensure the student's right to due process is maintained. Which of the following is not an appropriate step?

   A. The student is entitled to written notice of any charges against him or her.
   B. The student is provided sufficient opportunity to rebut the charges.
   C. The student has a right to an open hearing.
   D. The student has a right to have an adequate and accurate record of the proceedings.

3. Which of the following scenarios is appropriate regarding the use of peer feedback?

   A. The senior nurse learner is critiqued by the junior nurse learner on intravenous (IV)-line insertion.
   B. The learner at the same level evaluates his peer on a checklist worth 30% of the final grade.
   C. The peer provides feedback from an Objective Structured Clinical Examination (OSCE) that was done 6 weeks ago.
   D. The learner observes his peer inserting an indwelling catheter, then in privacy offers feedback regarding specific things done right or wrong.

4. Academic matters, as opposed to disciplinary matters, in clinical nursing education include:

   A. Threatening a student in class

   B. Fraternity or sorority curfew violation

   C. Harassing a student on Facebook

   D. Exhibiting uncontrolled anger in clinical

5. In order to facilitate socialization to the role of professional nurse, the clinical nurse educator focuses on creating a clinical learning environment conducive to the transition. Which activity best demonstrates this?

   A. Bringing snacks for the staff on the unit and having students write a thank-you note to them at the end of the rotation

   B. Asking a nurse or staff to pay extra attention to a weak nursing learner

   C. Appropriately adjusting the level of supervision provided to learners based on their needs

   D. Encouraging the nurse learner to assist the aide with emptying the patient's bedpan

6. A learner is struggling with care-plan sequencing in the clinical learning environment. The student tells the clinical nurse educator that he is a kinesthetic learner. The clinical nurse educator can best assist him to understand the nursing process by:

   A. Using a YouTube video

   B. Switching to a concept map

   C. Have the student role-play what a nurse would do

   D. Ask the student Socratic questions

7. Which activity would best foster learning and increase student learner satisfaction in the clinical environment?

   A. Assigning the student learner to observe the insertion of a peripherally inserted central catheter (PICC) line

   B. Talking through the rationale for withholding a medication

   C. Rotating the student learner to another floor

   D. Having the student write a paper on acute renal failure as a makeup assignment

8. What can the clinical nurse educator do to promote realistic student self-assessment?

   A. Make the self-assessment a percentage of the final grade.

   B. Point out student learner strengths, while minimizing weaknesses.

   C. Point out learner weaknesses to other students and staff.

   D. Provide truthful negative feedback in a nonjudgmental way.

9. What action would a clinical nurse educator take when a nursing student is grossly unsafe in the clinical environment?

A. Move the student off the clinical unit.

B. Coassign the student to another student.

C. Coassign the student to a nurse.

D. Provide an observational clinical experience.

10. The clinical nurse educator is new to the clinical learning environment (CLE). What could she do that would be most beneficial for the student learners?

A. Work part time on the unit so that she knows the "ins and outs" of the system.

B. Take the administrators out for a nice meal to "pave the way" for a smooth experience.

C. Set a tone of professionalism and respect for both staff and student learners.

D. Discuss the weaknesses of students with staff.

11. The clinical nurse educator wants to increase creativity in her student learners. What is the best way to achieve this?

A. Enroll in an art class.

B. Encourage divergent thinking through assignments and discussions.

C. Administer a med-math quiz.

D. Instruct the student learner to observe a Women, Infants, and Children (WIC) class at the local public health department.

12. In order to enhance learning, the clinical nurse educator should look for opportunities for the student learner to:

A. Give a report in bedside rounds.

B. Transport the patient to the radiology department.

C. Take a verbal order from the physician.

D. Observe the physical therapist perform range-of-motion exercises on the patient.

13. Which of the following scenarios correctly demonstrates the principle that student learners perform best when the level of supervision provided by the clinical nurse educator is appropriate to their needs?

A. The senior-level student learner who is assigned to a day in a rural clinic aspirates an effusion of the knee after receiving instruction from the nurse practitioner.

B. The junior-level student learner who has a child is assigned to provide discharge teaching for a new mom.

C. A junior-level student learner who has demonstrated proficiency in administering a medication via the subcutaneous route is instructed to administer medication via the nasal route with the help of a fellow student learner.

D. A senior-level student learner who has demonstrated proficiency in administering intramuscular (IM) injections is assigned to give flu shots at the flu clinic.

14. Which of the following demonstrates a trait in the clinical nurse educator that would most likely foster socialization to the role of nurse in the student learner?

A. Spends a majority of her day reviewing the electronic medical record (EMR) to ensure that documentation is accurate, thereby modeling the importance of accurate charting.

B. Builds trust by sharing details of her personal life.

C. Listens empathetically to a student learner's concerns about a clinical situation.

D. Encourages the student learner to conform to the practice of nurses on the unit by omitting steps in a procedure.

15. A nursing student is not progressing in the clinical environment as expected. She is not meeting the clinical objective related to comprehensive patient assessment, a previously learned competency/skill. The clinical nurse educator initially would:

A. Issue a clinical warning.

B. Issue a clinical failure.

C. Develop a learning contract.

D. Coassign the student to another student.

16. When asking learners to recall a medication's generic name, the clinical nurse educator is using what level of Bloom's taxonomy?

A. Understanding

B. Application

C. Comprehension

D. Analyzing

17. Recognizing that the complexity of healthcare today makes formal teaching of ethics to student learners more important than ever, the clinical nurse educator:

A. Advocates that the curriculum committee review the curriculum matrix, making sure ethics is addressed throughout the curriculum.

B. Suggests that clinical nurse educators share their moral opinions with students.

C. Reminds students about the tenets of the Nightingale Pledge.

D. Looks for ethical dilemmas in the clinical learning environment to involve students in.

18. When evaluating students' procedural knowledge about many different nursing interventions, the best evaluative mechanism is:

A. Objective structured clinical examination

B. Clinical skills checklist

C. Objective structured practical examination

D. Clinical rating scale

19. A student has not met the course expectations and requests an explanation. A good piece of evidence that demonstrates expectations would be:

A. Standards

B. Criteria

C. Course topical outline

D. Syllabus

20. The clinical nurse educator is not comfortable signing off on a student evaluation that the student works safely. This demonstrates what about the student?

A. The student learning outcomes

B. Understanding of the standards

C. Understanding of the evaluation process

D. Lack of competency

21. A comprehensive clinical evaluation plan consists of:

A. A formative and summative evaluation

B. Monthly performance objectives

C. Iterative feedback

D. Point-of-care feedback

22. A clinical nurse educator evaluates the students on the clinical evaluation scale throughout the academic term. The clinical nurse educator subscribes to a(n):

A. Analytical rubric

B. Totality assessment process

C. Holistic rubric

D. Formative process

23. The clinical nurse educator develops a plan with the student's involvement with 3 weeks left in the academic term. This constitutes:

A. Evaluation

B. Assessment

C. Guidelines

D. Remediation

24. Clinical preplanning for the clinical nurse educator includes:

A. Test construction

B. Review of the clinical evaluation tool

C. Develop the academic code of conduct

D. Review of new nurse orientation

25. When asking learners to explain a medication's side effect, the clinical nurse educator is using what level of Bloom's taxonomy?

    A. Understanding

    B. Application

    C. Comprehension

    D. Analyzing

26. The clinical nurse educator uses the faculty-made evaluation instrument and assesses each student in his clinical group against the rubric description. This is an example of:

    A. Assessment evaluation

    B. Norm-based evaluation

    C. Subjective evaluation

    D. Criterion-based evaluation

27. An effective evaluation tool used to assess students' clinical understanding of patient care when they cannot be present is:

    A. Case study

    B. Care plan

    C. Clinical skills checklist

    D. Clinical evaluation rubric

28. A nursing student makes a medication dosage error. The clinical nurse educator would:

    A. Acknowledge the error.

    B. Issue a clinical warning.

    C. Issue a failing grade.

    D. Report the student.

29. A clinical nurse educator faculty group is developing an evaluative instrument based on the course student learning outcomes (SLOs). This type of scale is most likely a:

    A. Case study

    B. Care plan

    C. Clinical skills checklist

    D. Clinical evaluation rubric

30. One method used to decrease the subjectivity of a clinical evaluation instrument is to:

    A. Add criteria.

    B. Measure specific competencies.

    C. Qualify the measures.

    D. Quantify the measures.

31. The goal of a clinical evaluation is to ensure:

    A. The student has passed the courses

    B. Ascertain what procedures have been completed

    C. Patient safety

    D. Promote NCLEX success

32. A clinical nurse educator would consider a student's repeated failure to turn in clinical assignments as:

    A. Lapsed behavior

    B. At-risk behavior

    C. Reckless behavior

    D. Knowledge-based behavior

33. Several nursing students approach the clinical nurse educator and inform her that a student is actively seeking and using opioids. The clinical nurse educator would take the following action:

    A. Allow the student to remain in the clinical area.

    B. Change the student's clinical experience to an observation experience.

    C. Report the student to the nurse manager.

    D. Confront the student about substance use.

34. The clinical nurse educator has a question regarding postclinical conference. She would consult which of the following?

    A. Course faculty/coordinator

    B. Department chair

    C. Dean

    D. Nurse manager

35. A nursing student nearing program completion reaches out to a professor whom she felt was well respected in the professional nursing community. The student asks the professor to serve as a preceptor to her as she enters the workforce. The professor explains to the student that she would help her more as a mentor versus a preceptor because:

    A. A mentor relationship is one that does not have to carry over into the working environment but can last for several years.

    B. It is a professional obligation for all new nurses to have mentors from nursing school in order to socialize appropriately into the workforce.

    C. A preceptor and a mentor are the same thing; however, professors can only serve as mentors.

    D. A preceptor and employee must sign a clinical contract for learning expectations and she cannot do this as a nonemployee at another facility or institution.

36. A nurse has recently completed her masters of science degree in nursing with a focus on education. She has worked as a bedside nurse on a medical–surgical nursing unit for the 3 years she has been a nurse and has been approached by her manager about being a unit-based educator for her peers, many of whom have been nurses for a much longer time than she has. In her new role, she finds that she is meeting resistance from her peers, who believe she is too young to be in the position. Her manager encourages her by reiterating the following statement regarding the nurse's clinical expertise:

   A. Her degree makes her the best person for the role.

   B. Clinical expertise is a combination of accumulated knowledge through experience, formal education, and use of evidence that guides clinical decision-making.

   C. Even if she does not have the years of nursing experience, this position will help her develop her clinical expertise.

   D. Nurses are known for "eating their young"; this is something she will just have to become accustomed to.

37. The nurse educator acknowledges that certification is important to her skill set because of which of the following?

   A. Certification increases salary.

   B. Certification is a requirement for clinical nurse educators.

   C. Certification is a method that clinical nurse educators use to validate their knowledge, skills, and experience beyond licensure.

   D. The clinical nurse educator certification is one that is intended for nurses working solely in academic settings.

38. The academic nursing program in which a nurse educator teaches does not focus on a single nursing theorist, but rather centers the curriculum around a combination of nursing theories. The educator learned *Orem's self-care deficit theory* as a nursing student and continues to exercise practice based on what she believes is derived from this theory. Which of the following concepts does she impress upon her students when caring for clients based on Orem's self-care deficit theory of nursing?

   A. Encourage the client to actively participate in all activities of daily living (ADL) that they can.

   B. Teach the family to do all care-related tasks for the client.

   C. Ensure nursing staff and assisting personnel are aware of client limitations and do not allow the patient to participate in care beyond this.

   D. Avoid use of interdisciplinary services such as occupational or physical therapy.

39. The nurse educator encourages her students to participate in leadership opportunities that will most likely help them enhance their future leadership potential. Which of the following activities would be least likely to serve as a springboard for opportunities in leadership in nursing?

   A. Act as the team leader during clinical days.

   B. Run for office in your academic program's student nurse association.

C. Join a nurses association in the state you plan to practice.

D. Participate in a journal club.

40. A learner is struggling with care-plan sequencing in the clinical learning environment. The student tells the clinical nurse educator that he is an auditory learner. The clinical nurse educator can best assist him to understand the nursing process by:

A. Using a YouTube

B. Switching to a concept map

C. Have the student role-play what a nurse would do

D. Ask the student Socratic questions

41. The nurse educator prepares an assignment for her clinical group. She asks the group to prioritize their patient list for rendering care. She instructs them to plan to assess the most critical patient first. What is the nurse educator trying to develop in the nursing student?

A. Personal growth

B. Cultural awareness

C. Clinical decision-making

D. Exploration and understanding of their own beliefs and values

42. A client admitted to a medical–surgical nursing floor has an implanted port that has been used to administer medications and obtain blood samples. The nurse educator demonstrates the process of obtaining a blood sample from the port to her students. The following week, the educator is notified that this patient has a double central line–associated bloodstream infection (CLABSI) and the hospital is performing a root cause analysis to determine a corrective action plan. The educator decides to share this scenario in a blind review as a case study with her students. She asks them to develop a mock action plan. What nursing skill is she trying to develop with these students?

A. Clinical reasoning

B. Correct process to draw blood

C. Learning to avoid being part of a legal proceeding

D. Learning when to avoid using implanted ports

43. The nurse educator prepares an assignment for her clinical group. She asks them to begin by developing a PICOT (patient/problem, intervention, comparison, outcome, time frame) question. She instructs them to learn the culture of the clinical unit and understand the patient population. Her desire is that they will, as a group, develop which of the following in order to give their project the momentum to achieve the best outcomes?

A. Personal relationships with the staff

B. Cultural awareness

C. A spirit of inquiry

D. Exploration and understanding of their own beliefs and values

44. The role of the clinical nurse specialist has changed and/or been eliminated over time largely due to a business model that ultimately eliminated the economic value of the role. Nursing has a large responsibility to advocate for this role because it supports client-driven outcomes that create positive health outcomes. This involves integrating best practices with which of the following?

    A. Clinical expertise and patient preference

    B. Personal experience and the clients' socioeconomic status

    C. Research utilization and policy review

    D. The nurses' experience and education level

45. Evidence demonstrates that students' satisfaction is increased when clinical nurse educators are:

    A. Personable to students

    B. Good delegators

    C. Organized

    D. Friendly with staff

46. The clinical nurse educator has a responsibility to balance student and patient needs. He or she can best do this by incorporating a model or set of competencies that create a framework for meeting these objectives. Which competency will help the educator balance her responsibilities?

    A. Value-based care

    B. Family-centered care

    C. Quality improvement

    D. Clinical preference

47. The clinical nurse educator is assisting students in performing health assessments and health histories. The primary objective for today's assignment is to develop the students' ability to obtain a more thorough and detailed focused assessment. The optimal method to teach then would be:

    A. Asking open-ended questions

    B. Asking yes or no questions

    C. Performing tests

    D. Seeing what the healthcare provider has documented

48. Discussing with students different viewpoints, perspectives, and ideas across disciplines is an ideal way to build:

    A. Cultural competence

    B. Collaboration

    C. Diversity

    D. Communication

49. Nursing students should be taught that evidence-based research has determined that using this skill reduces preventable healthcare errors:

A. Critical thinking

B. Collaboration

C. Self-reflection

D. Communication

50. It is imperative to reduce and eliminate incivility in the workplace, as it can create issues that impact both the staff and the patient. As the clinical nurse educator, you realize the main component to emphasize when educating students is:

A. Communication

B. Collaborative practice

C. Conflict management

D. Self-reflection

51. The clinical nurse educator is explaining to the clinical group that when one's values and ethics are not congruent with the organizations' values and ethics, a resulting effect may be:

A. Internal conflict

B. Organizational conflict

C. Personal alignment of their ethics to those of the organization

D. It does not create any conflict

52. An intrinsic factor that motivates clinical nurse educators to certification is:

A. Merit awards from employers

B. Rank promotion

C. Building confidence

D. Recognition by national organizations

53. While making rounds on the clinical nurse educator's assigned area, the clinical nurse educator brings a particular staff member to the clinical director's attention because this person has been engaging in inappropriate conversation with several healthcare providers. As the clinical nurse educator, you should:

A. Actively listen to environmental surroundings.

B. Remain calm.

C. Recognize conflict early.

D. Be proactive.

54. While conducting conflict management skill-building scenarios with your students, it is important to emphasize:

A. Utilize "you" statements.

B. Utilize "I" statements.

C. Place blame.

D. Avoid the situation.

55. It is essential for future professional nurses to develop this skill in order to effectively manage patient care through collaborative practice:

    A. Leadership

    B. Evidence-based practice

    C. Delegation

    D. Prioritization

56. Practicing collaboration builds on an important component(s), which is (are):

    A. Critical thinking

    B. Experience

    C. Quality and safety

    D. Trust and respect

57. While conducting strategies to resolve a conflict, a student member begins directing volatile comments at you. The best strategy for the clinical nurse educator to utilize is:

    A. Get up and leave.

    B. Return the volatile comments.

    C. Remain calm.

    D. Let someone else deal with this.

58. A student is talking at lunch about his family putting pressure on him to attend family events when he needs to be studying. What response by the clinical nurse educator would be most helpful?

    A. "Students usually have to put their social life on hold while in the nursing program."

    B. "You will need to tell your family that school is your priority now."

    C. "Tell your family that you are not feeling well and are unable to attend."

    D. "Let's talk about some time-management skills that may be helpful to you."

59. The clinical nurse educator notices that a student is quiet and isolated from the other students. After being asked whether anything was wrong, the student states that she feels that she has no connection to anyone and is questioning her career choice. What action by the clinical nurse educator would be most helpful?

    A. Send the student for counseling.

    B. Assign another student to work with her.

    C. Identify a mentor willing to work with the student.

    D. Recommend that she speak to a university guidance counselor.

60. A clinical nurse educator is using strategies to encourage clinical decision-making. What action by the educator would best facilitate this?

    A. Ask questions throughout the clinical day.

    B. Demonstrate skills before allowing students to perform them.

C. Provide explanations for complex patient care issues.

D. Encourage the students to observe the nurses in critical situations.

61. A clinical group is composed of eight multigenerational students. Which teaching–learning strategy would be most effective with this group?

   A. Lecture on a complex diagnosis during postconference.

   B. Assign a group project to be completed in postconference.

   C. Utilize a variety of methods based on student response.

   D. Require students to use smartphones to identify best practices.

62. One prominent reason there is an increased social need for clinical nurse educators is:

   A. There is an increased need for nurses due to baby boomers living longer.

   B. Nurses do not stay at the bedside.

   C. There are more second-degree nursing students who are older.

   D. Many clinical nurse educators team teach students.

63. A student informs her clinical nurse educator that the nurse she is working with is not answering questions and acts as though the student is an annoyance. How should the clinical nurse educator first respond?

   A. Remove the student from this nurse's assignment.

   B. Speak with the nurse manager about the nurse's behavior.

   C. Discuss student responsibilities with the nurse and her expectations.

   D. Question the student's interpretation of the nurse's behavior.

64. An experienced clinical nurse educator is describing the importance of facilitating the learners' understanding of the consequences of their actions following a simulation scenario. This technique is an example of:

   A. Active learning

   B. Reflective debriefing

   C. Constructive feedback

   D. Problem-solving

65. Students are found to be taking selfies with their smartphones in the nurses' station. Which response by the clinical nurse educator would be best in this situation?

   A. "This could be grounds for you all being dismissed from the nursing program."

   B. "You need to put away your phones before you are caught doing this."

   C. "You have been told that you cannot take pictures while in clinical."

   D. "This could be a breach of patient confidentiality if a name is seen in a picture."

66. A learner is struggling with care-plan sequencing in the clinical learning environment. The student tells the clinical nurse educator that he is a visual

learner. The clinical nurse educator can best assist him to understand the nursing process by:

A. Using a YouTube video

B. Switching to a concept map

C. Have him role-play what a nurse would do

D. Ask him Socratic questions

67. The clinical nurse educator overhears staff nurses laughing and disparaging a patient within hearing of several students. What is the educator's best response?

A. Ignore the behavior as harmless.

B. Inform the nurse manager of the incident.

C. Discuss the incident in postconference.

D. Confront the nurses about their behavior.

68. A novice clinical nurse educator tells her mentor that she works very hard to be tolerant of the differences of diverse individuals. What would be the mentor's best response?

A. "It is important to work toward embracing differences rather than tolerating them."

B. "Demonstrating tolerance is important in helping people to feel accepted."

C. "There are some students who are very difficult to like."

D. "You need to be fair to everyone so that no one feels discriminated against."

69. Following a patient code on the unit, students witness the clinical nurse educator assisting the unlicensed assistive personnel (UAP) to provide post-mortem care before the family arrives. This is an example of:

A. Mentoring the UAP

B. Educating the UAP

C. Modeling teamwork

D. Empathizing with the UAP

70. When asking learners to choose an intervention related to a medication's side effect, the clinical nurse educator is using what level of Bloom's taxonomy?

A. Understanding

B. Application

C. Comprehension

D. Creating

71. Many nurses learned about nursing care through on-the-job training. The type of learner who learns best with hands-on experience through clinical practice uses what type of learning style?

A. Visual learner

B. Audio learner

C. Kinesthetic learner

D. Multimodal learner

72. Clinical nurse educators who use a pedagogical approach to facilitate learners in an active style of teaching expect the students to:

A. Become involved in doing and thinking about what they are doing.

B. Participate in lecturing in the class.

C. Be diligent in taking notes in class.

D. Be ready to look up answers on their smartphones while listening in class.

73. Clinical nurse educators know working in the clinical setting can be very stressful for students. One method the nurse educator can use to reduce that stress and enhance student learning is to do which of the following?

A. Leave the unit and let the floor nurse monitor the student's activities.

B. Use humor appropriately and mindfulness training prior to patient care.

C. Allow the student to work more autonomously.

D. Allow the student to make small mistakes and correct them in postconference.

74. The clinical nurse educator will be bringing a new group of students to a new clinical site. The nurse educator realizes the students will have enhanced learning under which of the following conditions?

A. The nursing staff works closely with the faculty and is aware of the learning outcomes.

B. The nursing staff were former graduates of the school of nursing and know what to expect.

C. The nurse educator is completely in control of all nursing student activities.

D. Nursing staff only assign to students those patients who pose no real challenge to cause any disruptions in healthcare.

75. Clinical nurse educators who teach in the clinical setting realize evidence-based research is essential to teaching students how to:

A. Focus on critical thinking and clinical reasoning.

B. Never deviate from hospital-approved clinical pathways.

C. Always consult the clinical protocols before performing a procedure.

D. Consider using the tried-and-true methods of healthcare treatments.

76. Clinical nurse educators know critical thinking skills enhance the students' abilities to do which of the following?

A. Process information, problem-solve, and make judgments.

B. Know what to do in any given situation all the time.

C. Create a care plan that can be used universally for most patients.

D. Follow the same routine daily without deviation.

77. A clinical setting is conducive to learning when the student is able to do which of the following?

    A. Work independently without interference from the staff.

    B. Work with the staff who accepts the student with a positive attitude.

    C. Have an opportunity to meet the staff at an informal greeting outside of the clinic.

    D. Have relatives who work in the healthcare profession at another clinic.

78. The clinical nurse educator is teaching a group of students about cultural competence. The students understand what cultural competence is when:

    A. The student mimics someone else's culture and practices to make that person feel at home.

    B. The student asks the patient to explain why the patient believes in that culture.

    C. The student understands the unique needs and preferences of ethnic minorities without changing his or her own beliefs.

    D. The student expects others to change to follow current local customs now that they are no longer in their country.

79. Clinical nurse educators are always interested in bringing in new technology and strategies to teach students. Which of the following would be considered an active method of teaching to enhance clinical competencies?

    A. Have a guest speaker who is an expert in his or her field present to the class.

    B. Have the students participate in a field trip to a specialized clinic to observe new experiences.

    C. Incorporate simulation-based clinical experiences for the student in a controlled and safe environment.

    D. Have the students present previously learned clinical experiences in class.

80. Which of the following is the best assignment to help learners use evidence-based practice to improve clinical safety?

    A. Ask learners to identify a safety issue in clinical practice and have them research evidence-based practices related to this issue.

    B. Ask learners to read an article about clinical safety and evidence-based practices.

    C. Show the learners a video about clinical safety and evidence-based practices.

    D. Lead a class discussion about clinical safety and evidence-based practices.

81. Which of the following is considered an intrinsic motivator that could be the reason why a candidate is seeking certification?

    A. Maintaining employment

    B. Career advancement

    C. Financial incentive

    D. Sense of accomplishment

82. The nurse educator has asked learners to do a concept map of a patient's care plan but finds that some learners are having difficulty creating this map. Which type of learner is most likely to construct a well-created map?

    A. Visual

    B. Kinesthetic

    C. Auditory

    D. Read/Write

83. The benefit of evaluating learners in the learning lab and in clinical settings is the ability to evaluate which type of learning?

    A. Cognitive

    B. Psychomotor

    C. Affective

    D. Moral

84. Which is an accurate statement related to studying within a group?

    A. No leader should be identified in order to be sure all group members are considered equal.

    B. There should be a start time but the study session should continue until all learners feel it is time to stop.

    C. Breaks should be taken whenever the learners feel overwhelmed or fatigued.

    D. Establish a set topic to discuss that day with clear outcomes expected.

85. What cognitive level from Bloom's taxonomy does the following question fit: "You have just received your patient's electrolyte results and note the potassium is 3.2 mEq/L. What nursing interventions are needed?"

    A. Knowledge

    B. Application

    C. Analysis

    D. Evaluation

86. When one experiences test anxiety, a coping strategy to employ would be to have the person:

    A. Arrive at the testing center 5 minutes before the test begins to avoid hearing others talk about the exam.

    B. Perform a last-minute review the evening prior to the scheduled exam.

    C. Carry out deep-breathing techniques and use guided imagery.

    D. Tell yourself that you have never been a great test-taker and not to expect the best.

87. It is the evening before the candidate's scheduled exam. What would be the most beneficial way to spend this evening?

    A. Go out to a nightclub for drinks and dancing with friends.

    B. Stay up as late as possible to continue studying his or her weak content areas.

    C. Spend the evening at home with family watching movies.

    D. Spend time on the phone talking to a friend who is complaining about her boyfriend.

**88.** The clinical nurse educator is role-modeling the importance of interprofessional communication and collaboration while on the clinical unit. Which National League for Nursing (NLN) core competency is this nurse educator exhibiting?

    A. Functioning as a change agent and leader

    B. Pursuing continuous quality improvement in the nurse educator role

    C. Engaging in scholarship

    D. Facilitating learner development and socialization

**89.** Which of the following statements is true related to the Certified Academic Clinical Nurse Educator (CNE®cl) certification examination?

    A. Every question on the examination counts toward your overall score.

    B. It is composed mainly of low-level thinking items because it emphasizes specific details.

    C. Items are written by a select few nurse educators coming from one type of program located within a small geographic range.

    D. It relies heavily on forming associations among various concepts and applying knowledge in a contextual manner.

**90.** The best method for the clinical nurse educator to use to validate her or his skills is to:

    A. Develop policies and procedures.

    B. Contribute to didactic test questions.

    C. Work as staff on the unit where he or she teaches.

    D. Obtain certification.

**91.** A student states that he believes that a patient's cancer was caused by environmental chemicals. The clinical nurse educator asks the student to describe the type of cancer and then to make the link from the environmental chemical to the pathology. This type of coaching can be considered:

    A. Direct questioning

    B. Reflection

    C. Scaffolding

    D. Care planning

**92.** The clinical nurse educator has a good understanding of student preparedness when he states:

    A. "I will ask them to discuss their patients in preconference."

    B. "I will administer a quiz before they start the day."

C. "The staff nurse will tell them what they need to know for their patients."

D. "Only the patient's main diagnosis should be addressed in the care plan initially."

93. When dealing with a student who fails the clinical practicum, a novice clinical nurse educator needs additional understanding of "due process" when she states:

A. "I have provided the student with a warning about her poor performance before the failure."

B. "The student should understand that she has been consistently performing poorly."

C. "The student did not follow the plan for improvement as signed."

D. "The student was told on multiple occasions that without improvement this would be a course failure."

94. The novice clinical nurse educator needs additional understanding of evidence-based clinical teaching practice when he states:

A. "The acute care center that is Magnet recognized may offer more learning opportunities."

B. "I have made sure that all students are at the same place each semester for continuity."

C. "The 'nursing home' is not a good place for students to learn skills."

D. "Assessing the culture of the clinical environment is important for learning opportunities."

95. One method of ensuring that students have the most up-to-date evidence to base their patient care decisions on in the clinical learning environment (CLE) is to use:

A. Textbooks that are less than 5 years old

B. Journal articles less than 5 years old

C. The healthcare organization's policies

D. A mobile app designed for reference

96. One of the reasons for high attrition rates for graduate nurses is:

A. Lack of physical skill attainment

B. Decreasing pay scales

C. Overmentoring

D. Lack of ability to make judgments

97. A method to assist the novice clinical nurse educator fulfill the role is to:

A. Have the educator take an academic nursing education course.

B. Provide the educator with a mentor.

C. Tell the educator to use her or his clinical experience as a guide.

D. Instruct the educator to match the students with staff nurses.

98. An undergraduate nursing student passes out in the clinical area and is not hurt. The staff tell the clinical nurse educator that she did not eat. The clinical nurse educator should first:

    A. Provide her with a snack.

    B. Call her parents to come get her.

    C. Have her taken to the emergency room.

    D. Notify the course coordinator.

99. The novice clinical nurse educator needs better understanding of the concept of *integrity* when he identifies that integrity involves:

    A. Honesty

    B. Ethical behavior

    C. Role-modeling

    D. Professionalism

100. An effective method used to teach students leadership in the clinical learning environment (CLE) is:

    A. Have them shadow the nurse manager.

    B. Have them create assignments.

    C. Ask them to teach a group of patients.

    D. Have them role-model being in charge.

# 12

## Posttest Questions and Answers

### ANSWERS AND RATIONALES FOR CHAPTER 2

1. The clinical nurse educator observed that students were struggling with normal lab values. She creates an electronic Jeopardy game using brief scenarios to enhance their knowledge base. This teaching strategy would be most effective for which type of learner?

   A. Visual—NO, prefer charts, diagrams, symbols, and pictures.

   B. Auditory—NO, prefer teaching concepts to others within a study group.

   **C. Kinesthetic—YES, prefer using virtual simulations, role-playing, or gaming.**

   D. Read/Write—NO, prefer writing notes in the margins to highlight important points.

2. The examination candidate should make which content area a priority as it accounts for 19% of the exam items?

   **A. Facilitate Learning in the Healthcare Environment—YES, comprises 19% of exam.**

   B. Facilitate Learner Development and Socialization—NO, comprises 15% of exam.

   C. Implement Effective Clinical Assessment and Evaluation Strategies—NO, comprises 17% of exam.

   D. Apply Clinical Expertise in the Healthcare Environment—NO, comprises 15% of exam.

3. On the day of the examination, which would be the most nutritious food choice for the candidate to consume?

   A. Bran muffin and a soy latte with two shots of expresso—NO, avoid caffeinated beverages that could increase anxiety and interrupt learning.

   B. Two chocolate eclairs with a glass of whole milk—NO, chocolate contains caffeine and is a refined sugar, which can sap energy quickly.

   **C. Whole wheat bagel and a fruit smoothie with kale—YES, complex carbohydrates (CHO), fruits, and vegetables are ideal to fuel the mind and body.**

   D. Cheese omelette with an orange energy drink—NO, while the eggs are high in protein, the energy drink can induce or increase existing anxiety.

4. Which of the following is an example of surface learning?

   A. Making links between concepts—NO, this is an example of deep learning.

   **B. Memorizing facts, figures, and tables—YES, this is surface learning and usually occurs when one is cramming for an examination at the last minute.**

   C. Relating current material to previously learned material—NO, this is an example of deep learning.

   D. Organizing information into categories—NO, this is an example of deep learning.

5. After the learners witnessed a code blue in progress during their clinical day, the clinical nurse educator asks the learners to write a self-reflective journal describing their experience. According to Bloom's taxonomy, which domain of learning is best being evaluated?

   A. Cognitive—NO, although it takes thought to write a self-reflective journal, this is not the best method to use in evaluating this domain.

   **B. Affective—YES, this is a technique that allows the learners to discuss their feelings and emotions regarding the situation.**

   C. Psychomotor—NO, there is no actual carrying out of procedures/skills.

   D. Comprehension—NO, this is one of six cognitive levels of thinking.

6. The clinical nurse educator develops a case study for the learners to complete during a postconference. One of the requirements is for the learner to create a teaching plan for the patient. Which of the following cognitive levels is being asked of the student?

   A. Knowledge—NO, it involves recall and would not be useful to individualize a teaching plan.

   B. Application—NO, this expects the learner to implement an intervention to a problem.

   C. Analysis—NO, this includes the ability of the learner to understand why a solution was effective or not.

   **D. Synthesis—YES, this provides the opportunity to bring all concepts together and design a plan to create solutions to problems.**

7. Which of the following demonstrates an effective method of studying?

   **A. Answering practice questions that mimic the actual certification exam, including environment and time frame—YES, this will increase your confidence level when it is time to take the certification exam.**

   B. Identifying the tricks and strategies of the examination to reduce the amount of material that needs to be studied—NO, there is no magic bullet in taking the exam as it is testing essential concepts, which you need to have learned.

   C. Read only the rationales to questions you answered incorrectly while taking practice exams—NO, it is important to read all rationales to every question as it can provide information to potentially help you answer similar, subsequent questions on that topic.

   D. Study only when time allows within your schedule—NO, if you do not set up a realistic study plan, it is too easy to become distracted and procrastinate.

8. Which eligibility criteria must be met to sit for the Certified Academic Clinical Nurse Educator (CNE®cl) certification examination and is found in both options?

   A. A baccalaureate degree in nursing—NO, this is found only in Option A.

   B. Two years of teaching experience in an academic setting within the past 5 years—NO, this is found only in Option A.

   C. A graduate degree with a focus on nursing education—NO, this is found only in Option B.

   **D. Three years in any area of nursing practice—YES, this is a requirement for both Option A and B.**

9. A candidate fails her certification exam the first time she sits for it. She asks whether she can reapply to retake the exam. What is the best response to provide to her?

   A. "No, since you have taken it and were unsuccessful, there is no chance to retake."—NO, a candidate is able to retake the exam but needs to wait a minimum of 90 days to reapply.

   B. "Yes, you can retake the exam but you must sit for a remediation course before you can reapply."—NO, there is no statement indicating that a candidate must sit for a remediation course prior to retaking the certification exam. This candidate should use the information provided to identify strengths and weakness to perform better next time.

   **C. "Yes, you can retake the exam in 90 days but cannot exceed taking the exam four times within a year."—YES, a candidate can reapply to sit for the exam but must wait the 90 days before reapplying. This wait time is a great opportunity to continue studying especially on the topics they identified as weaknesses.**

   D. "No, because you have seen the questions on the exam and it would not be a fair assessment of your actual performance."—NO, there is a large pool of questions; therefore, the chances of getting the identical exam is slim to none. Candidates do have the opportunity to retake once the 90 days has elapsed.

10. A clinical nurse educator, who took and passed the exam 6 years ago, continues to use the credential Certified Academic Clinical Nurse Educator (CNE®cl) after her name. When asked whether she has renewed her certification, she denies doing so. What would be the best response by the director of the nursing program in which she is employed?

   A. "You can continue to use those credentials; however, please renew this certification as soon as possible."—NO, the certification is only valid for 5 years so the credentials can no longer be used until successful recertification has been carried out.

   B. **"You are not permitted to use those credentials any longer since it is only valid for 5 years and you must retake the examination since you allowed the certification to expire."—YES, once the 5-year period has elapsed, the credentials can no longer be used. Since this clinical nurse educator allowed her certification to expire, she will have to reapply (pending meeting the new eligibility criteria) to sit for the examination.**

   C. "It is fortunate for you that one does not have to renew this certification."—NO, renewal is required and must be done every 5 years.

   D. "Since you are currently in a teaching position and you are assigned to a clinical practicum with students, recertification is not required."—NO, despite being in clinical with students, this does not automatically renew one's certification. There is a process to abide by.

## ▨ ANSWERS AND RATIONALES FOR CHAPTER 3

1. An elderly patient admitted with a urinary tract infection is demonstrating deterioration in his status. When speaking to the patient's student nurse, the clinical nurse educator discusses her own assessment of the situation and rationales for further interventions. This is an example of

   A. Psychomotor apprenticeship—NO, apprenticeship is learning through the observation of physical skills.

   B. **Cognitive apprenticeship—YES, learning occurs through observation of the expert's thinking processes.**

   C. Socratic questioning—NO, this is questioning that encourages a deeper level of thinking from the learner.

   D. Autocratic leadership—NO, this is a style of leadership that allows little input from others.

2. A new clinical nurse educator is relating to his mentor how he coached a student today. What statement would indicate that the educator needs further information on coaching?

   A. "My student observed me providing instructions on insulin administration today."—NO, this is an example of modeling.

   B. "Instead of directly answering questions, I had my student look up the answer."—NO, this would be an example of the student searching for the evidence.

   C. "I required my student to explain the rationale for each of her interventions."—NO, this is an example of articulation when using cognitive apprenticeship.

D. "I observed my student perform her assessment and then I provided feedback."—YES, observation followed by individualized feedback is an example of coaching.

3. An experienced clinical nurse educator is working to better motivate her students. How can the educator influence the student who is extrinsically motivated?

A. **Assign a letter grade as part of the feedback on concept maps.—YES, those who are extrinsically motivated usually perform in order to achieve high grades.**

B. Praise the student after completing new skills.—NO, intrinsically motivated students respond best following positive feedback.

C. List areas for improvement following a procedure.—NO, neutral or negative feedback alone does not usually serve as a motivator.

D. Assign a challenging dressing change that the student has performed previously.—NO, a sense of accomplishment is more effective if intrinsically motivated.

4. A clinical nurse educator expresses to her mentor an interest in using debriefing in postconferences. Which statement by the clinical nurse educator indicates an accurate understanding of the debriefing process?

A. "Debriefing is a simple process that can be done in a few minutes."—NO, the learners must be provided adequate time to allow for reflection; this is usually more than a few minutes.

B. "Debriefing focuses on highlighting all that was done incorrectly by the student."—NO, the purpose is to guide students to connect their actions to the outcomes.

C. "During the debriefing, I will be reflecting on what could have been done differently."—NO, the students should be involved in self-reflection.

D. **"In order to be effective with my debriefing, I will first seek training opportunities."—YES, it is very important that whomever is debriefing has received adequate training.**

5. Students have been assigned to keep a reflective journal of their clinical experiences. What statement by the novice clinical nurse educator would indicate that further instruction is needed relative to the reflective journals?

A. "It is important that a trusting relationship be developed so students will feel safe in documenting their feelings."—NO, if the students do not feel safe, they are more likely to write what they believe the educator wants to hear.

B. **"Changes in attitudes should be noted early in the reflective journaling process."—YES, learners must be given time for reflection; change occurs over time.**

C. "When reading their journals, it is important to remain nonjudgmental."—NO, this is important for students to feel safe in sharing their honest feelings.

D. "Students need instruction on the purpose and benefits of reflective journaling."—NO, in providing a reason and benefit for the activity, students are more likely to engage in self-reflection.

6. A clinical nurse educator is planning an assignment that will promote leadership skills. Which assignment would be most effective?

   **A. Instruct the student to delegate non-nursing tasks to the unlicensed assistive personnel.—YES, delegation is an effective use of leadership skills.**

   B. Assign the student to observe the charge nurse for the day.—NO, observation is a much less effective way of learning.

   C. Assign the student to perform complete care for the patient.—NO, this does not require the student to use leadership skills.

   D. Inform the student he will be administering medications to his patient today.—NO, this does not require the student to use leadership skills.

7. A nurse manager is overheard talking about students being on their phones in the clinical learning environment (CLE). What action by the clinical nurse educator would be least helpful in this situation?

   A. Check the agency policy to ensure students are not in violation.—NO, this would be appropriate to ensure that no policy is being violated.

   B. Meet privately with the nurse manager to address her concerns.—NO, this would be the most direct method of determining the nurse manager's concerns.

   **C. Inform the nurse manager that this is the future of technology in practice.—YES, although this statement may be true, it could serve to further inflame the situation.**

   D. Monitor the students' phone usage to ensure they are not on social media.—NO, the clinical nurse educator should monitor student usage to ensure the device is not being accessed for unauthorized use.

8. A clinical nurse educator is talking to a colleague about the use of mobile devices in the clinical learning environment (CLE). Which statement provides the best argument for its use?

   **A. "Students have access to a multitude of references allowing them to search for the current, best evidence."—YES, this actively involves students in identifying best practice.**

   B. "Students and faculty can continue to access email and remain connected to their courses and instructors."—NO, this is not an important use of technology in practice and has the potential of being misused.

   C. "The professional nursing staff are constantly using their phones, so there is no reason the students shouldn't as well."—NO, this is not a valid reason for students to use mobile devices.

   D. "Students are more engaged when they are using their phones and working as a team."—NO, using mobile devices in the CLE runs the risk of isolating the user and making them less aware of their surroundings.

9. A clinical nurse educator is trying to ensure inclusive excellence in the clinical learning environment (CLE). What action would be most effective in achieving this?

A. Ask all students in postconference to discuss their ethnic background.—NO, this is not appropriate or effective.

B. Require all students to speak up during postconference activities.—NO, this may make some students extremely uncomfortable.

C. **Provide students with the opportunity to speak openly and freely in postconference.—YES, this creates an environment of trust and respect where students feel safe to speak.**

D. Invite a minority nurse to speak to the students in postconference.—NO, this would not help to create an environment of inclusiveness.

10. A student is observed sitting at the nurse's station using a smartphone while call lights are ringing. What would be the best response for the clinical nurse educator?

A. Take the student's phone for the remainder of the clinical day.—NO, smartphones are personal property and should not be taken from the student, although they can be instructed to put it away.

B. **Privately meet with the student to discuss appropriate use of the smartphone.—YES, a discussion on prioritization and quality patient care would be appropriate.**

C. Inform the student that she will be receiving a clinical warning.—NO, this is an extreme response for a first-time offense; start with educating the student.

D. Prohibit smartphone use in the clinical learning environment (CLE) for the rest of the semester.—NO, this is an extreme response that would impact the entire clinical group.

## ▪ ANSWERS AND RATIONALES FOR CHAPTER 4

1. The academic clinical educator plan to do an educational activity to have the learners demonstrate postoperative assessment techniques. Which activity will be the most effective?

A. Case study report of a postoperative patient—NO, this is not the best assignment.

B. **Simulation activity using the human patient simulator—YES, this is an excellent way for the learner to demonstrate an assessment.**

C. Literature review of postoperative care—NO, this is not the best assignment.

D. Computer simulation of a postoperative patient—NO, this is not the best assignment.

2. The academic clinical educator wants to evaluate the therapeutic communication of the learners. Which activity will be the most effective?

A. Case study report of a postoperative patient—NO, this is not the best assignment.

B. **Simulation activity using a standardized patient—YES, using a standardized patient is an excellent way to assess therapeutic communication.**

C. Literature review of therapeutic communication—NO, this is not the best assignment, it is passive.

D. Computer simulation of a postoperative patient—NO, this is not the best assignment, because simulation may be more realistic.

3. Which of the following can be implemented during orientation to a new clinical site to best reach the goal of familiarizing students with the type of patients on the unit?

A. Treasure hunt—NO, this is a good way to familiarize students to the clinical learning environment (CLE).

B. Electronic Medication Records training—NO, this is needed but will not familiarize students with the patient population.

C. **Review of medical records and documentation—YES, this will speak to the patient population.**

D. Introducing students to patients—NO, this will only superficially familiarize the students with the patient population.

4. Which of the following techniques includes clarifying questions to help determine the best approach?

A. Case studies—NO, this will assist with decisions in the case, but may or may not be applicable to the clinical learning environment (CLE).

B. Problem-based learning—NO, this is also good for didactic decision-making about clinical issues.

C. **Reflective learning—YES, reflective learning includes the use of clarifying questions to obtain additional information.**

D. Socratic questioning—NO, this leads students to reflective thinking.

5. The best explanation a clinical nurse educator can provide students about TeamSTEPPS® is

A. An analysis process used by individuals in the clinical setting—NO, this does not capture its essence.

B. A research process used for evidence-based practice (EBP)—NO, it uses EBP but is not a process to develop EBP.

C. **A teamwork system developed by the Agency for Healthcare Research and Quality—YES, it is to improve team functioning.**

D. A teamwork EBP process developed by the Agency for Healthcare Research and Quality—NO, it was not developed for research purposes.

6. The clinical nurse educator understands that a student who is reluctant to call the primary care provider about a needed medication change should be

A. Instructed to leave the unit because the student is unprepared—NO, this means that they need to be remediated on this particular skill.

B. Remediated about TeamSTEPPS®—NO, this is an interprofessional approach but may not be most effective for this situation.

C. Provided with a clinical warning and a learning plan—NO, although a learning plan is appropriate, a remediation would increase the student's confidence.

**D. Taken to the simulation laboratory for practice—YES, practice is the best remediation to increase the student's confidence.**

7. A novice nurse educator states that electronic medical records (EMR) should be taught after students learn how to document longhand because that is the way she learned and it was useful. The best recommendation to the novice nurse educator is to

A. Tell her that longhand documentation is outdated.—NO, this does not provide the clinical nurse educator the best rationale.

B. The school only uses EMR documentation.—NO, this is not the best rationale to provide.

C. She should explain both methods to students.—NO, this is not what the faculty of the nursing program has decided.

**D. She should participate in the skills laboratory when students are being orientated to documentation.—YES, this will assist the clinical nurse educator to understand what is being taught and why to the students.**

8. A novice nurse educator assigns students to specialty units for multiple days during the medical course. The course instructor should review with the novice educator

**A. The student learning outcomes for the course—YES, the observations must meet the student learning outcomes.**

B. The skills the students should know—NO, skills are not as important as the student learning outcomes that encompass both theory and skills.

C. The old clinical schedules—NO, these are not the most helpful for the novice to understand the rationale.

D. Her philosophy of hands-on education—NO, this may not be well developed if this is her first clinical group.

9. Dedicated Education Units (DEUs) have improved learner outcomes by

A. Having learners do evidence-based projects—NO, this is not done universally.

B. Reassigning the same patients to students—NO, this is not always possible.

**C. Having a consistent, educated preceptor—YES, preceptors who are experienced are often knowledgeable about teaching/learning strategies as well as policies/procedures in the CLE.**

D. Having independence in the student role—NO, there is a preceptor.

10. Congruency in clinical placement to the adult-gerontology healthy aging course would be

A. An acute care facility—NO, this is not representative of healthy aging.

B. A long-term care facility—NO, this is not representative of healthy aging.

C. Outpatient facility—NO, this is not representative of healthy aging.

**D. Adult day care—YES, this is a better representation of healthy adult aging.**

## ▨ ANSWERS AND RATIONALES FOR CHAPTER 5

1. The clinical nurse educator is conducting preconference and a junior nursing student is unable to answer questions about her assigned patient's diagnosis or safety concerns. The clinical nurse educator should:

   **A. Send the student off the clinical unit.—YES, the student is not safe without knowledge.**

   B. Coassign the student to another student nurse.—NO, the student is not safe without knowledge.

   C. Assign the student to a nurse.—NO, the student is not safe without knowledge.

   D. Issue a clinical failure for the course.—NO, the student requires due process.

2. The clinical nurse educator learns that a student in her clinical group is working a full-time night shift and going to an accelerated nursing program full time. The clinical nurse educator should:

   A. Do nothing as the student's work schedule is not the school's concern.—NO, this is a safety concern.

   **B. Inform the student in writing that she needs to follow the policy related to consecutive nursing hours.—YES, lack of sleep is a safety concern.**

   C. Allow the student to begin clinical at a later time.—NO, the student has the same start time as other students and could still be a safety concern.

   D. Call the student's employer.—NO, the clinical nurse educator would not interfere with a student–employee relationship.

3. The clinical nurse educator issues a learning contract to her nursing student for which purpose?

   A. In order to award a clinical warning—NO, this is not the purpose of a learning contract.

   B. To protect he faculty against litigation—NO, this is not the purpose of a learning contract.

   **C. To assist student in meeting the clinical objectives—YES, this is the purpose of a learning contract.**

   D. In order to award a failing grade—NO, this is not the purpose of a learning contract.

4. The focus of the remediation plan should be to:

   **A. Support student learning and mastery of competencies.—YES, this is the focus of remediation.**

   B. Document clinical deficiencies.—NO, this is not the focus of remediation.

C. Protect the faculty member against litigation.—NO this is not the focus of remediation.

D. Acknowledge students' clinical competence.—NO, this is not the focus of remediation.

5. Due process, as it applies to clinical nursing education, is described as:

A. Procedural safeguards that are established in protection of patient safety—NO, this is not due process with respect to the student in the clinical environment.

B. Procedural safeguards that are established in protection of academic honesty—NO, this is not due process with respect to the student in the clinical environment.

C. Procedural safeguards that are established in protection of student privacy—NO, this is not due process with respect to the student in the clinical environment.

D. **Procedural safeguards that are established on how issues of academic misconduct or performance will be treated**—YES, this is due process as it applies to clinical education.

6. "Just culture" applied to clinical nursing education is described as:

A. Critical incident debriefing is held with the nursing staff.—NO, this is not "just culture" in clinical education.

B. **Students learn and improve by openly identifying and examining their weaknesses.—YES, this is "just culture" as it applied to clinical education.**

C. Students attend all required remediation sessions.—NO, this is not "just culture" in clinical education.

D. Students can question the clinical nurse educator.—NO, this is not "just culture" in clinical education.

7. Reckless behavior for students engaged in a clinical practicum would include:

A. Arriving late to clinical—NO, this is not reckless behavior.

B. Reporting positive information to the clinical nurse educator—NO, this is not reckless behavior.

C. Failing to follow the chain of command—NO, this is not reckless behavior.

D. **Lack of clinical preparation—YES, this is reckless behavior and can harm the patient.**

8. A student misreads a medication label on a busy medical–surgical floor resulting in a near-miss medication error. This type of error is described as:

A. **Human error—YES, this is an example of a human error due to a lapse or slip.**

B. At-risk error—NO, this is not at-risk behavior.

C. Reckless error—NO, this is not reckless behavior.

D. Rule-based error—NO, there is no category for high-risk error.

9. If a nursing student engages in abusive, "bullying" behaviors, the clinical educator would consider this behavior as:

A. Lapsed behavior—NO, this is not a human error.

B. At-risk behavior—NO, this is not at-risk behavior.

C. **Reckless behavior—YES, this is a reckless behavior that can cause harm to patients.**

D. Skill-based behavior—NO, there is no category for high-risk behavior.

10. If a student looks up or discusses private information about patients outside of specified patient assignment/responsibilities, this behavior would be considered:

A. Human error—NO, this is not a human error.

B. At-risk behavior—NO, this is not at-risk behavior.

C. **Reckless behavior—YES, this is reckless behavior that can harm a patient.**

D. Knowledge-based behavior—NO, there is no category for high-risk behavior.

## ▦ ANSWERS AND RATIONALES FOR CHAPTER 6

1. Clinical nurse educators should consider using various methods of teaching. According to visual, aural/auditory, read/write, and kinesthetic (VARK) learners, which learning style enjoys listening to tape recording and problem-solving?

A. Visual learners—NO, the learners with this learning style prefer visuals.

B. Kinesthetic learners—NO, these learners like hands-on learning.

C. Multimodal learners—NO, these learners have more than one dominant learning style and can move from one to another.

D. **Audio learners—YES, student with this learning type like to hear content and instructions.**

2. To meet the learning needs of the student, the clinical nurse educator will need to develop several strategies for teaching. Which of the following strategies would best demonstrate the model of education that meets the needs of the student?

A. **Student centered—YES, this provides student engagement.**

B. Group centered—NO, not all students learn best in groups.

C. Nursing centered—NO, students are many times just learning to think like a nurse.

D. Educator centered—NO, this is more about the clinical nurse educator's needs.

3. The nurse educator is collecting data to analyze information that can improve instruction and student learning while it is happening. Which of the following best explains this type of assessment?

A. Summative assessment—NO, this is done at the end and often comes with a grade.

B. **Formative assessment—YES, this provides the student with a plan for improvement.**

C. Diagnostic assessment—NO, this is not usually a learning term.

D. Impact assessment—NO, this is not usually a learning term.

4. The nursing faculty and administration plan to make a major change in the curriculum for the nursing program. The department realizes the current status quo will be destabilized. According to Lewin's theory of change, which stage of change would be occurring at this time?

A. **Unfreezing—YES, this is the stage that starts the change process and disrupts status quo.**

B. Movement—NO, this happens after the unfreezing.

C. Refreezing—NO, this solidifies the changes.

D. Debriefing—NO, this lets people reflect on learned content or changes.

5. Which of the following could be considered a nursing theory that promotes and helps the student become self-sufficient?

A. **Self-care—YES, this promotes caring for oneself so nurses can care for others.**

B. Self-aware—NO, this is not a theory.

C. Autocratic—NO, this is a leadership style.

D. Reliant—NO, this is not a theory and students are taught not to rely on others but to be self-reliant.

6. In the quality improvement of education, which of the following would the clinical nurse educator include in the clinical experiences?

A. **Best evidence—YES, this promotes quality care.**

B. Past experiences—NO, this may not have been on a professional level for students.

C. Recent events—NO, this may not be the best way to inform care.

D. Local customs—NO, this may not be the best way to inform care.

7. Nursing turnover can be very costly to the administration. One way to reduce that turnover is to provide nursing mentors. Which of the following best demonstrates the purpose and end result of having a nursing mentor?

A. **As a retention strategy—YES, there is evidence to demonstrate there is a reduction in nurses leaving the bedside.**

B. A relationship builder—NO, this is not the best method.

C. A best friend—NO, this is not evidence based.

D. A career guide—NO, this is not evidence based.

8. Clinical evaluations and assessment data are kept for many reasons. Which of the following explains the best reason for keeping these data?

A. **They help to determine the achievement of the student.—YES, this documents learning of content and skills.**

B. They encourage the students' progress in the course.—NO, that would be a formative evaluation.

C. They allow others to see how a great educational program is taught.—NO, that is not the main purpose.

D. Emphasizes the experience the clinical nurse educator demonstrates—NO, that is not the purpose.

9. The nursing department is advertising for a clinical nurse educator to help redesign the clinical component of the curriculum. Which of the following type of clinical nurse educator would have the skills to create and articulate a positive change?

A. Someone with good people skills—NO, this is helpful but not the main attribute needed.

B. Someone with very high personal integrity—NO, this is helpful but not the main attribute needed.

C. **Someone with a great strategic vision—YES, the person needs to be able to understand the needs of the faculty, students, and community.**

D. Someone with excellent technical skills—NO, this is helpful but not the main attribute needed.

10. The clinical nurse educator is evaluating a student who is having difficulty understanding basic concepts presented in the clinical learning environment. Which of the following would be the first step the nurse educator should take to help this student?

A. Enroll the student in a remediation course.—NO, this may not be available.

B. Send the student to the student learning center for evaluation.—NO, this may be a good second step.

C. **Have the student take a visual, aural/auditory, read/write, and kinesthetic (VARK) test to see what learning style the student has.—YES, this may be a good first step to see whether it is simply a difference in learning styles.**

D. Have the student study with a group of senior students.—NO, this may not help.

## ▨ ANSWERS AND RATIONALES FOR CHAPTER 7

1. The clinical nurse educator observes a student not coming forward with needed, pertinent information to a team member from another discipline. The clinical nurse educator should:

A. Remove the student from the situation.—NO, this does not assist the student in learning from the situation.

B. Tell the student to talk with the team member privately.—NO, this does not assist the student in evaluating what needs to be learned in order to develop this skill.

C. **Assist the student in developing this skill.—YES, it is important to assess where the student is currently, develop strategies, and establish practice sessions to develop the skill.**

D. Discuss this situation with the student.—NO, although it is important to discuss what is happening with the student at the present time, it is important to assess and implement strategies to build this skill.

2. The clinical nurse educator observes and hears a nursing student say, "It is not my job to clean the soiled patient, it is the unlicensed assistive personal's responsibility." The clinical nurse educator should:

A. Discuss this situation in postconference.—NO, it is important to discuss this issue, but the topic needs to be broadened out to discuss teamwork, without singling out a particular person.

B. Find a private moment and a place to talk with the student one on one.—NO, this may be appropriate, but the other students will not learn the appropriate responses.

C. Let this matter go for now because he or she is a good student.—NO, the student will not learn about the concept and the importance of teamwork.

D. **Discuss roles and responsibilities, teamwork, and resolutions with the group.—YES, it is important for the entire clinical group to learn about the importance of teamwork.**

3. The clinical nurse educator is with a student administering medications through a comatose patient's nasogastric tube. The student is explaining everything to the patient. A medical resident is also present in the room and observes this. The medical resident asks: "Why are you talking to the patient, he is comatose?" The clinical nurse educator should:

A. Speak with the medical resident's superior.—NO, it is important to pass the information on, so the medical residence can work on respectful communication. However, the student will not learn how to properly handle this type of situation.

B. **Role model the correct conflict response with the student present.—YES, it is important to role-model in front of the student the proper way to deal with conflict.**

C. Confront the medical resident without the student present.—NO, the student will not learn the proper way to handle conflict.

D. Pull the medical resident aside later and talk to her about the comment.—NO, the student will not learn the proper way to handle conflict and the student still may think this is ok.

4. As the clinical nurse educator, several healthcare providers have come to you to say that the new group of nursing students is not providing appropriate and relevant information when queried by the nursing staff. You have completed your assessment of the situation and determined that:

A. A debriefing should be done with the students—NO, debriefing is utilized after an incident to determine what worked well, what did not, and what needs to be changed to prevent reoccurrence.

B. Conflict resolution should be conducted between the staff and the health-care providers.—NO, even though this has created conflict for the health-care providers, there is a lack of communication created by lack of knowledge and skill.

C. **Educate/reeducate the students on utilizing SBAR (situation, background, assessment, and recommendation).—YES, it is important to educate/reeducate the new graduates on the use of the communication tool, SBAR.**

D. Educate/reeducate the students on collaborative practice.—NO, even though collaborative practice is important, providing correct, detailed, pulled together information is needed.

5. The performance assessment of a procedure you witnessed on one of your assigned nursing floors is being done by two of your students; the assessment is chaotic and has no direction. As the clinical nurse educator, you realize:

A. You should provide additional procedural education and training.—NO, additional education and training may be needed, but the proper tool at this moment is utilizing debriefing to find out the viewpoint of the students.

B. **Establish debriefing to discuss what went well and what did not.—YES, debriefing is needed to obtain the viewpoint of the students of what worked well, what did not work well, and what can be done to improve the process and outcome.**

C. Allow the students some time to collect themselves.—NO, even though work needs to continue and the students may need to calm down, they do need to discuss their emotions and thoughts through debriefing.

D. Have the students retake the fundamentals-of-nursing course.—NO, the staff may need to review the steps; however, the best alternative would be to do practice drills.

6. The Joint Commission, American Nurses Association, and other organizations have determined this to be a core competency that begins at the baccalaureate level:

A. Advocacy for the nursing profession—NO, even though this is of importance, this is not a core competency.

B. Delegation and prioritization—NO, it is important to possess this skill set. However, it is not a core competency.

C. Performing quality-improvement projects—NO, it is important to possess knowledge of these categories; however, this is not a core competency.

D. **Communication and collaboration—YES, these are core competencies that are also listed as core competencies in *The Essentials of Baccalaureate Education for Professional Nursing Practice.***

7. As you are making rounds on your assigned floor, you encounter several nursing students discussing a situation that occurred this week. You realize you need to implement conflict management. One of the most important skills you need to use is:

A. **Listening—YES, this is one of the most important skills to possess in conflict management.**

B. Building trust—NO, this is an important skill, however, listening is primary.

C. Understanding group dynamics—NO, even though this is important, the primary skill to utilize is listening.

D. Understanding educational dynamics—NO, even though this is important, the primary skill to utilize is listening.

8. It is time for postconference and you notice that several of the students are not communicating with each other and you sense tension in the air. As the clinical nurse educator you should:

   A. Just let this past, they will work this out for themselves.—NO, it is important to be vigilant for impending conflict and act proactively.

   B. Not become involved, pass this on to the course coordinator.—NO, it is important to be proactive now before this conflict continues to escalate.

   C. **Establish a conflict-management implementation.—YES, conflict resolution needs to begin now before it escalates.**

   D. Manage your uncomfortable emotions.—NO, even it is important to be self-reflective and calm, a resolution must begin now.

9. An important concept and key component for nursing students to grasp and carry throughout their lifelong learning that is crucial in all aspects of communication is to develop:

   A. Leadership skills—NO, this is an important skill to have now in today's healthcare environment; however, a key component is self-reflection.

   B. Communication skills—NO, this is an important skill to have now in today's healthcare environment; however, a key component is self-reflection.

   C. Conflict-management skills—NO, this is an important skill to have now in today's healthcare environment; however, a key component is self-reflection.

   D. **Self-reflection skills—YES, this skill is needed to understanding oneself and one's reactions to situations.**

10. A student says: "I do not understand why you are making me go and talk to this person that I do not get along with in our clinical group, when you should be handling the situation." As the clinical nurse educator, you reply:

    A. "What makes you feel that way?"—NO, it is important to let students voice their sides, but does not create accountability for solving the issue. If this statement is used, it must be reflected back to the student learning about conflict management.

    B. "You are the one accountable for your relationship."—NO, this is not the best answer. If this statement is used, it must be reflected back to the student learning about conflict management.

    C. **"Remember, you need to develop your conflict-resolution skills."—YES, this is the best answer to remind the student to take accountability, and to practice this skill set.**

   D. "Avoidance is not going to make your problem go away."—NO, even though this is a true statement, it is not the best answer to reflect back to the student.

## ▪ ANSWERS AND RATIONALES FOR CHAPTER 8

   1. The clinical nurse educator assesses the clinical decision-making skills of the student by which means?

      A. Care plan review—NO, this is a part of the paperwork submitted.

      B. Concept maps—NO, this does not necessarily assess decision-making.

      C. Debriefing—NO, this is a time for reflecting on what was learned.

      **D. Bedside questioning—YES, bedside questioning is an active strategy for assessing students' skills.**

   2. Which of the following is considered in the integration of care in evidence-based practice (EBP)?

      **A. Patient preference—YES, this is considered in the integration of care.**

      B. Family preference—NO, it is an influence but not considered in the integration.

      C. Expert opinion—NO, it is an influence but not considered in the integration.

      D. Physician expertise—NO, it is an influence but not considered in the integration.

   3. What is the first step in the evidence-based practice (EBP) process?

      A. Ask the clinical question—NO, this is the second step.

      **B. Spirit of inquiry—YES, questioning the status quo is the first step.**

      C. Collect the most relevant evidence—NO, this is the third step.

      D. Critically appraise the evidence—NO, this is the fourth step.

   4. Which leadership characteristic of the clinical nurse educator involves demonstrating best practice?

      A. Mentoring—NO, this involves building a relationship and establishing goals.

      B. Precepting—NO, this involves developing specific outcomes for the inexperienced nurse to perform in a specified time.

      **C. Role modeling—YES, educators demonstrate best clinical practice and professional behavior when role-modeling.**

      D. Personal attention—NO, this is the attitude of the nurse educator as she develops into her role.

   5. Which strategy helps develop clinical expertise?

      **A. Use real-life scenarios—YES, this strategy helps students recognize real situations and how to respond.**

      B. Administer content tests—NO, this tests didactic knowledge.

    C. Concept maps—NO, these are used to assess clinical information.

    D. Review case studies—NO, this uses passive action that does not develop clinical skills.

6. The doctor of nursing practice (DNP) degree trains nurses to become proficient in what area?

    A. Identify new procedures.—NO, this is not an identified area.

    **B. Evaluate evidence-based practices for care.—YES, identified by the National Organization of Nurse Practitioner Faculties (NONPF).**

    C. Research for breakthroughs.—NO, this is not an identified area.

    D. Develop interdisciplinary standards.—NO, this is not an identified area.

7. Which is the most effective tool for the clinical faculty member to use to teach concept mapping to a group of fundamentals-level nursing students?

    **A. Review of exemplars from senior-level nursing students—YES, exemplars will aid with grasping and understanding the concept for new students.**

    B. Review of the clinical facility electronic health record (EHR) care plan—NO, care plans in the electronic health record are standardized interventions that are not always relevant for the individual patient.

    C. Review completed concept maps during postconference.—NO, reviewing the students' work is effective, but for novice nursing students, it is often more helpful to review examples of other students who have effectively grasped concept mapping.

    D. Begin with teaching about creating a linear care plan—NO, not effective for teaching.

8. Senior nursing students are asked to submit a topic for approval for an evidence-based practice project that they can implement on their clinical unit. Which student submission will be given back to the student for further clarification before proceeding with the project?

    A. Decreased use of indwelling Foley catheters decrease the incidence of catheter-associated urinary tract infections.—NO, a feasible project.

    B. Appropriately timed collection of stool samples from patients with suspected *Clostridium difficile* infection in order to correctly identify or rule out a hospital-acquired infection.—NO, a feasible project.

    C. The use of scheduled mouth care for mechanically ventilated patients decreases the incidence of ventilator-associated pneumonia.—NO, a feasible project.

    **D. Biphasic defibrillators decrease the incidence of code blue situations in an acute care setting.—YES, needs more specific information to demonstrate a relationship.**

9. The clinical course coordinator is planning student–preceptor assignments for an upcoming semester by reviewing former student evaluations of nurse preceptors on a medical–surgical unit. When evaluating to determine whether or not preceptors would be asked to precept subsequent students, the clinical faculty finds which of the following is helpful in making concrete decisions about inviting preceptors to continue precepting students?

A. The students make comments about relationships formed with the preceptor outside of work/school—NO, this reflects personal opinion.

B. **The student's use of hospital policy and practice standards when performing new skills with the preceptor—YES, demonstrates evidence-based practice.**

C. The student's feedback on the complexity of patients being more than a student should care for while still a student—NO, this is the opinion of individual.

D. The student's opinion of how the unit is managed by the nurse manager—NO, this is opinion, not fact.

10. With the shift to many clinical nurse specialists (CNS) assuming supervisory roles in practice settings, which of the following job-related responsibilities is likely not to have been included in a traditional clinical nurse specialist academic program of study?

A. Role of change agent—NO, this is a CNS role.

B. Role of a leader—NO, this is a CNS role.

C. **Role of manager—YES, this is not a role of the clinical nurse specialist.**

D. Role of clinical expert—NO, this is a CNS role.

## ■ ANSWERS AND RATIONALES FOR CHAPTER 9

1. The student asks the clinical nurse educator to eat dinner with the clinical group at a restaurant. The clinical nurse educator should:

A. Accept the invitation but only stay for 30 minutes.—NO, the clinical nurse educator is still joining them for a social outing.

B. Decline with no explanation.—NO, the clinical nurse educator should explain the rationale to the students.

C. **Tell the students that it is better that they go to dinner by themselves.—YES, the clinical nurse educator should maintain boundaries between himself or herself and students.**

D. Suggest a restaurant with a band and bar.—NO, it is not appropriate to drink alcohol with students.

2. The clinical nurse educator has received a social media "friend" request from a student. What should the clinical nurse educator tell the student?

A. I would love to connect with you on social media.—NO, accepting "friend" requests may interfere with professional boundaries.

B. **I must decline your request in order to maintain faculty–student boundaries.—YES, the clinical nurse educator should maintain boundaries by declining "friend" requests with students.**

C. I cannot be your "friend" on social media while you are in this course, but you can ask me in a later semester.—NO, it is not ideal to accept "friend" requests from current students, even if they are not in your current course.

D. I only accept "friend" requests from students who have As in the course.—NO, this reflects favoritism of the clinical nurse educator toward certain groups of students.

3. A nursing student wears a hijab due to her Muslim religion. What does the clinical nurse educator tell her in the clinical learning environment?

   A. You must remove your hijab while in clinical. It is not part of your nursing uniform.—NO, it is possible to accommodate other cultural practices while in the clinical learning environment.

   B. You may wear your hijab, but only if you explain it to each patient.—NO, the student is not required to explain her hijab and religion to each patient.

   C. **You may wear your hijab in clinical. I know that it is an important part of your religion.—YES, the student should be allowed to wear a hijab since it is an important part of her religion.**

   D. You need to quit wearing your hijab because I am concerned about infection control.—NO, the clinical nurse educator should not require the student to stop wearing the hijab. The student may continue to follow all infection-control practices while wearing the hijab.

4. The clinical nurse educator wants to encourage active learning in the postclinical conference. Which of the following would indicate that the clinical nurse educator needs additional instruction in active learning strategies?

   A. **Lecture the students about the most common diagnoses encountered in the clinical learning environment.—YES, lecture is not an active learning strategy, so the clinical nurse educator would need additional instruction.**

   B. Have each student present information about his or her patient.—NO, this strategy engages student actively.

   C. Assign students a presentation topic for postclinical conference.—NO, this strategy encourages the active involvement of students and promotes leadership skills.

   D. Play an educational game that relates to the diagnoses in the clinical learning environment.—NO, games actively engage students so this is an appropriate active learning strategy.

5. Which of the following would indicate that a nursing student needs additional instruction on self-care?

   A. **I get 3 hours of sleep each night.—YES, this student needs to be instructed about the importance of adequate sleep as a part of self-care.**

   B. I eat a healthy diet.—NO, a healthy diet is a part of self-care.

   C. I exercise for 30 minutes three or four times per week.—NO, a regular exercise is a part of self-care.

   D. I meditate each day.—NO, medication and spirituality are a part of self-care.

6. The clinical nurse educator hears a nursing student talking about how stressful the nursing program is. Which statement by the clinical nurse educator is most appropriate?

A. **Mindfulness-based stress reduction can help with stress relief.—YES, this is an evidence-based stress-reduction technique.**

B. You have to learn to live with the stress. It will only get worse once you are a nurse.—NO, this is not a therapeutic statement. The clinical nurse educator needs to suggest a stress-reduction strategy to the student.

C. I use energy drinks to cope with stress.—NO, this is not an evidence-based strategy to decrease stress.

D. I try to just do the tasks for each patient and try not to connect emotionally with patients.—NO, it is important for nurses to provide high-quality, compassionate care to patients and not just accomplish tasks. This is not an appropriate stress-reduction strategy.

7. A nursing student turns in a concept map that is similar to another student's concept map. What is the best response by the clinical nurse educator?

A. You worked with your classmate, and teamwork is important in nursing.—NO, plagiarism must be addressed in the clinical learning environment.

B. Your patients had the same diagnoses, so I understand why your concept maps look similar.—NO, plagiarism of another student's work must be addressed by the clinical nurse educator.

C. **Plagiarism is not acceptable in the clinical learning environment.—YES, it is important that students are aware that plagiarism is not allowed in the classroom or the clinical learning environment.**

D. The concept map is not graded. In the future, be sure to turn in your own work.—NO, plagiarism is not acceptable even on ungraded work.

8. The clinical nurse educator is concerned that a student is exhibiting incivility when the student engages in which activity?

A. The student looks up the patient's medications on a smartphone application (app).—NO, it is appropriate for the student to look up medications on an approved smartphone app.

B. **The student texts a friend about dinner plans.—YES, this behavior is incivil because it does not pertain to the clinical learning environment.**

C. The student asks the primary nurse about the time of a scheduled procedure.—NO, the student is asking the nurse about the patient's procedure time so that nursing care can be planned.

D. The student requests permission to observe the wound care nurse's evaluation of his patient.—NO, the student desires to learn more by observing the wound care nurse at work.

9. Which of the following is the best way to encourage active learning about the quality-improvement process?

A. Give a quiz on quality improvement during postclinical conference.—NO, this does not encourage active learning about quality improvement.

B. **Encourage student participation in quality-improvement projects in the clinical learning environment.—YES, this encourages students to learn about the quality-improvement process in the clinical learning environment.**

    C. Lecture on quality improvement during postclinical conference.—NO, this is not an active learning strategy.

    D. Give students an article on the Quality and Safety Education in Nursing competencies.—NO, this is not an active learning strategy.

10. A clinical nurse educator is providing an orientation to new nursing students. The educator encourages students to join one of the nursing student organizations on campus. How will joining an organization assist students to be successful in the nursing program?

    **A. Encourages students to socialize to the role of the nursing student.—YES, joining an organization may assist with socialization to the role of the nursing student.**

    B. Teaches job-searching skills.—NO, this is not the main purpose of nursing student organizations.

    C. Reviews anatomy and physiology content.—NO, this is not the main purpose of nursing student organizations.

    D. Permits students to go on trips to conferences.—NO, this is not the main purpose of nursing student organizations, although some organizations do sponsor trips to conferences.

## ■ ANSWERS AND RATIONALES FOR CHAPTER 10

1. A clinical nurse educator is reviewing a student's care plans, concept maps, and anecdotal notes about the student to inform him of a grade. The clinical nurse educator is making a(n):

    A. Judgment—NO, he is actually using evidence to make an assessment.

    B. Evaluation—NO, he is actually using evidence to make an assessment.

    **C. Assessment—YES, he is collecting evidence.**

    D. Remediation plan—NO, there is no indication this is for process improvement.

2. The clinical nurse educator grades all the students' care maps in the clinical group and places them in a pile from best to worst and assigns grades. This a an evaluation process known as:

    A. Assessment evaluation—NO, because a grade is being assigned.

    **B. Norm-based evaluation—YES, the students are being ranked.**

    C. Subjective evaluation—NO, the clinical nurse educator is using a ranking system.

    D. Criterion-based evaluation—NO, the clinical nurse educator is not comparing the assessment to criteria.

3. Clinical nurse educators understand that the clinical evaluation process needs further research to develop better:

    A. Validity—NO, content validity is done on every developed tool by expert opinion.

    **B. Reliability—YES, is it reliable group after group.**

    C. Assessment skills—NO, clinical nurse educators know how to evaluate assessment skills.

    D. Criteria—NO, clinical nurse educators understand what criteria need to be meet for a professional nurse due to established standards.

4. The clinical nurse educator is developing a rubric for the students' care maps. The clinic nurse educator is placing a value for each component of the map on the rubric. The clinical nurse educator is making a(n):

    A. Criterion—NO, the clinical nurse educator is making a judgment or evaluation of each criteria on the rubric.

    **B. Evaluation—YES, the clinical nurse education is making a judgment.**

    C. Assessment—NO, the clinical nurse educator is making a judgment or evaluation of each criteria on the rubric.

    D. Remediation plan—NO, this is a formative evaluative process.

5. Regulatory and professional nursing organizations help establish:

    **A. Competencies and standards—YES, for public safety.**

    B. Assessments for grading—NO, they are not prescriptive.

    C. Safe and unsafe behavior indicators—NO, they are not that specific.

    D. Pass/fail criteria—NO, they do not make such judgments.

6. One of the advantages of evaluating clinical learning experiences compared to classroom processes is the ability to evaluate:

    A. Cognitive learning—NO, both can evaluate critical thinking.

    **B. Psychomotor learning—YES, this is a hands-on learning environment.**

    C. Affective learning—NO, this also can be evaluated in the classroom by professionalism.

    D. Procedural learning—NO, this is just one piece of psychomotor learning.

7. When using Objective Structured Clinical Examinations (OSCEs) for high-stakes evaluation, it is most important that the clinical nurse educator ensures:

    A. The students are prepared.—NO, although this is an important piece.

    B. The faculty understand the processes.—NO, although this, too, is needed.

    **C. The conditions are standardized.—YES, or the evaluation process is not fair.**

    D. The standardized patients used display the symptoms.—NO, this is not always necessary or feasible.

8. The clinical nurse educator is using her anecdotal notes at midterm to debrief a student about an improvement process. The clinical nurse educator is developing a:

    A. Summative evaluation—NO, this assigns an end-of-term grade.

    **B. Formative evaluation—YES, this is a process-improvement mechanism.**

    C. Pass/fail decision—NO, this is summative.

    D. Course grade—NO, this is also summative.

9. The clinical nurse educator is using the total assessment material at the end of the semester to assign a pass/fail grade to a student. The clinical nurse educator is developing a(n):

   A. **Summative evaluation—YES, this is done at the end of the semester.**

   B. Formative evaluation—NO, this allows for process improvement.

   C. Remediation plan—NO, this allows for process improvement.

   D. Assessment—NO, this is not the judgment needed for evaluation.

10. A clinical nurse educator is reviewing the standards for the clinical learning environment (CLE) and finds them broad in scope. The clinical nurse educator should next review the:

    A. Student learning outcomes (SLOs)—NO, these may not match up exactly with standards for the CLE.

    B. **Criteria—YES, these break down the standards to be more specific.**

    C. Course topical outline—NO, these topics may not match up exactly with standards for the CLE.

    D. Syllabus—NO, this may only have the general SLOs.

## ▪ ANSWERS AND RATIONALES FOR PRACTICE TEST

1. A clinical nurse educator waits until the end of the academic term to evaluate the students on their clinical performance. She subscribes to a(n):

   A. Analytical rubric—NO, this is used for individual assignments.

   B. **Totality assessment process—YES, this can be used for final or summative grades.**

   C. Holistic rubric—NO, this means it is done all at once.

   D. Formative process—NO, this is usually an evaluation for process improvement.

2. When misconduct failures or dismissals are enacted, several steps must be taken by the clinical faculty to ensure the student's right to due process is maintained. Which of the following is not an appropriate step?

   A. The student is entitled to written notice of any charges against him or her.—NO, this is an appropriate step.

   B. The student is provided sufficient opportunity to rebut the charges.—NO, this is an appropriate step.

   C. **The student has a right to an open hearing.—YES, this is the correct response as the hearing does not have to be open to the public.**

   D. The student has a right to have an adequate and accurate record of the proceedings.—NO, this is an appropriate step.

3. Which of the following scenarios is appropriate regarding the use of peer feedback?

A. The senior nurse learner is critiqued by the junior nurse learner on intra-venous (IV)-line insertion.—NO, this would likely be unhelpful and could make both learners uncomfortable.

B. The learner at the same level evaluates his peer on a checlist worth 30% of the final grade.—No, this is not an appropriate use of feedback.

C. The peer provides feedback from an Objective Structured Clinical Exam-ination (OSCE) that was done 6 weeks ago.—NO, feedback should be given as close to the time of the activity as possible so that improvements can be made.

**D. The learner observes his peer inserting an indwelling catheter, then in privacy offers feedback regarding specific things done right or wrong.— YES, this is appropriate.**

4. Academic matters, as opposed to disciplinary matters, in clinical nursing edu-cation include:

A. Threatening a student in class—NO, this is a disciplinary matter.

B. Fraternity or sorority curfew violation—NO, this is a disciplinary matter.

C. Harassing a student on Facebook—NO, this is a disciplinary matter.

**D. Exhibiting uncontrolled anger in clinical—YES, this is an academic mat-ter in a clinical program.**

5. In order to facilitate socialization to the role of professional nurse, the clinical nurse educator focuses on creating a clinical learning environment conducive to the transition. Which activity best demonstrates this?

A. Bringing snacks for the staff on the unit and having students write a thank-you note to them at the end of the rotation—NO, this may help create a pleasant environment, but does not assure that the environment is foster-ing socialization to the role.

B. Asking a nurse or staff to pay extra attention to a weak nursing learner—NO, this does not help create a good clinical learning environment.

**C. Appropriately adjusting the level of supervision provided to learners based on their needs—YES, providing the appropriate level of supervi-sion has been shown to promote socialization to the role.**

D. Encouraging the nurse learner to assist the aide with emptying the patient's bedpan—NO, this is important to know how to do but does not help with socialization to the role.

6. A learner is struggling with care-plan sequencing in the clinical learning envi-ronment. The student tells the clinical nurse educator that he is a kinesthetic learner. The clinical nurse educator can best assist him to understand the nursing process by:

A. Using a YouTube video—NO, this would better suit a visual learner.

B. Switching to a concept map—NO, this would better suit a visual learner.

**C. Have the student role-play what a nurse would do—YES, this would assist a kinesthetic learner.**

D. Ask the student Socratic questions—NO, this would better suit an audi-tory learner.

7. Which activity would best foster learning and increase student learner satisfaction in the clinical environment?

   A. Assigning the student learner to observe the insertion of a peripherally inserted central catheter (PICC) line—NO, providing opportunities for students to engage in skills offers better experiences.

   **B. Talking through the rationale for withholding a medication—YES, teaching clinical reasoning is beneficial.**

   C. Rotating the student learner to another floor—NO, an available clinical nurse educator provides the best experience.

   D. Having the student write a paper on acute renal failure as a makeup assignment—NO, this does not teach clinical reasoning or allow the student to engage in clinical skills.

8. What can the clinical nurse educator do to promote realistic student self-assessment?

   A. Make the self-assessment a percentage of the final grade.—NO, this could cause inflated self-assessment.

   B. Point out student learner strengths, minimizing weaknesses.—NO, this could cause inflated self-assessment.

   C. Point out learner weaknesses to other students and staff.—NO, this is demeaning and could set up a defensive response in the learner.

   **D. Provide truthful negative feedback in a nonjudgmental way.—YES, this helps the student gain an understanding of the expected benchmark and gives permission for the expression of areas needing improvement.**

9. What action would a clinical nurse educator take when a nursing student is grossly unsafe in the clinical environment?

   **A. Move the student off the clinical unit.—YES, this is correct as patient safety is a priority.**

   B. Coassign the student to another student.—NO, this is not correct as this action jeopardizes patient safety.

   C. Coassign the student to a nurse.—NO, this is not correct as this action jeopardizes patient safety.

   D. Provide an observational clinical experience.—NO, this is not correct as the student has been unsafe and requires consequences.

10. The clinical nurse educator is new to the clinical learning environment (CLE). What could she do that would be most beneficial for the student learners?

    A. Work part time on the unit so that she knows the "ins and outs" of the system.—NO, this may or may not be helpful.

    B. Take the administrators out for a nice meal to "pave the way" for a smooth experience.—NO, this type of behavior does not lead to better clinical experiences.

    **C. Set a tone of professionalism and respect for both staff and student learners.—YES, staff and student learners will respond to this and be more likely to work well together.**

D. Discuss the weaknesses of students with staff.—NO, this does not enhance the CLE.

11. The clinical nurse educator wants to increase creativity in her student learners. What is the best way to achieve this?

A. Enroll in an art class.—NO, although it is important to enhance the clinical nurse educator's own creativity, this may not necessarily increase creativity in student learners.

B. **Encourage divergent thinking through assignments and discussions.— YES, this is an acceptable way of increasing creative thinking.**

C. Administer a med-math quiz.—NO, although a necessary skill, this does not enhance creativity.

D. Instruct the student learner to observe a Women, Infants, and Children (WIC) class at the local public health department.—NO, although important information is gleaned from this activity, it does not necessarily foster creative thinking.

12. In order to enhance learning, the clinical nurse educator should look for opportunities for the student learner to:

A. **Give a report in bedside rounds.—YES, this is the best choice because it engages the student learner as part of the healthcare team.**

B. Transport the patient to the radiology department.—NO, this does not engage the student learner.

C. Take a verbal order from the physician.—NO, a student learner should never do this.

D. Observe the physical therapist perform range-of-motion exercises on the patient.—NO, this does not engage the student.

13. Which of the following scenarios correctly demonstrates the principle that student learners perform best when the level of supervision provided by the clinical nurse educator is appropriate to their needs?

A. The senior-level student learner who is assigned to a day in a rural clinic aspirates an effusion of the knee after receiving instruction from the nurse practitioner.—NO, this is not appropriate or within the scope of practice.

B. The junior-level student learner who has a child is assigned to provide discharge teaching for a new mom.—NO, the student does not necessarily have the required knowledge for this.

C. A junior-level student learner who has demonstrated proficiency in administering a medication via the subcutaneous route is instructed to administer medication via the nasal route with the help of a fellow student learner.—NO, the clinical nurse educator should oversee this.

D. **A senior-level student learner who has demonstrated proficiency in administering intramuscular (IM) injections is assigned to give flu shots at the flu clinic.—YES, this is appropriate.**

14. Which of the following demonstrates a trait in the clinical nurse educator that would most likely foster socialization to the role of nurse in the student learner?

A. Spends a majority of her day reviewing the electronic medical record (EMR) to ensure that documentation is accurate, thereby modeling the importance of accurate charting.—NO, attending is the desired trait.

B. Builds trust by sharing details of her personal life.—NO, this is inappropriate and does not maintain healthy boundaries.

C. **Listens empathetically to a student learner's concerns about a clinical situation.—YES, empathy is a desired trait.**

D. Encourages the student learner to conform to the practice of nurses on the unit by omitting steps in a procedure.—NO, this does not foster learning or socialization to the role.

15. A nursing student is not progressing in the clinical environment as expected. She is not meeting the clinical objective related to comprehensive patient assessment, a previously learned competency/skill. The clinical nurse educator initially would:

A. Issue a clinical warning.—NO, this is not correct as the student needs an opportunity to improve.

B. Issue a clinical failure.—NO, this is not correct as the student needs an opportunity to improve.

C. **Develop a learning contract.—YES, a learning contract provides the student an opportunity to improve.**

D. Coassign the student to another student.—NO, the student is not in a position to supervise another student.

16. When asking learners to recall a medication's generic name, the clinical nurse educator is using what level of Bloom's taxonomy?

A. **Understanding—YES, this is recall only.**

B. Application—NO, the question is not asking for an intervention.

C. Comprehension—NO, the question is not asking to solve an issue.

D. Analyzing—NO, the question is not asking the learner to organize or compare and choose an action.

17. Recognizing that the complexity of healthcare today makes formal teaching of ethics to student learners more important than ever, the clinical nurse educator:

A. **Advocates that the curriculum committee review the curriculum matrix, making sure ethics is addressed throughout the curriculum.—YES, this is one way that enhances ethical comportment in student learners.**

B. Suggests that clinical nurse educators share their moral opinions with students.—NO, this is not the best way.

C. Reminds students about the tenets of the Nightingale Pledge.—NO, ethical practice is based on the American Nurses Association's (ANA) *Code of Ethics.*

D. Looks for ethical dilemmas in the clinical learning environment to involve students in.—NO, this is not the best way to teach ethics.

18. When evaluating students' procedural knowledge about many different nursing interventions, the best evaluative mechanism is:

A. Objective structured clinical examination—NO, this is usually based on just one encounter.

B. Clinical skills checklist—NO, this just demonstrates whether and how well a skill was performed.

**C. Objective Structured Physical Examination—YES, because typically there are stations to address.**

D. Clinical rating scale—NO, this usually addresses standards and criteria or student learning outcomes (SLOs).

19. A student has not met the course expectations and requests an explanation. A good piece of evidence that demonstrates expectations would be:

**A. Standards—YES, standards are expectations of a professional nurse.**

B. Criteria—NO, criteria describe the standards, which are the overall expectations.

C. Course topical outline—NO, this is what will be taught didactically.

D. Syllabus—NO, this is about the course expectations.

20. The clinical nurse educator is not comfortable signing off on a student evaluation that the student works safely. This demonstrates what about the student:

A. The student learning outcomes—NO, these are general standards.

B. Understanding of the standards—NO, the student may understand but the behavior may not display that understanding.

C. Understanding of the evaluation process—NO, this should not be a factor.

**D. Lack of competency—YES, if the student is not safe alone.**

21. A comprehensive clinical evaluation plan consists of:

**A. A formative and summative evaluation—YES, this is a comprehensive evaluation plan.**

B. Monthly performance objectives—NO, this is only one aspect of a clinical evaluation.

C. Iterative feedback—NO, this is only one aspect of a clinical evaluation.

D. Point-of-care feedback—NO, this is only one aspect of a clinical evaluation.

22. A clinical nurse educator evaluates the students on the clinical evaluation scale throughout the academic term. The clinical nurse educator subscribes to a(n):

**A. Analytical rubric—YES, this process does not evaluate all standards at once.**

B. Totality assessment process—NO, this is not the process.

C. Holistic rubric—NO, this evaluates all standards at the end.

D. Formative process—NO, this is a process that allows process improvement.

23. The clinical nurse educator develops a plan with the student's involvement with 3 weeks left in the academic term. This constitutes:

    A. Evaluation—NO, this is the end evaluative process.

    B. Assessment—NO, this is gathering evidence to make a judgment.

    C. Guidelines—NO, these are standards.

    **D. Remediation—YES, this assists the student to improve.**

24. Clinical preplanning for the clinical nurse educator includes:

    A. Test construction—NO, this is not part of clinical preplanning.

    **B. Review of the clinical evaluation tool—YES, this is part of clinical pre-planning for the clinical nurse educator.**

    C. Develop the academic code of conduct—NO, this is not part of clinical preplanning.

    D. Review of new nurse orientation—NO, this is not part of clinical preplanning.

25. When asking learners to explain a medication's side effect, the clinical nurse educator is using what level of Bloom's taxonomy?

    A. Understanding—NO, this is recall.

    B. Application—NO, this is translating knowledge into practice.

    **C. Comprehension—YES, this understands what something does or does not do.**

    D. Analyzing—NO, this is taking information and sorting and choosing from it.

26. The clinical nurse educator uses the faculty-made evaluation instrument and assesses each student in his clinical group against the rubric description. This is an example of:

    A. Assessment evaluation—NO, this is collecting data.

    B. Norm-based evaluation—NO, this is ranking students' performance.

    C. Subjective evaluation—NO, this is being judgmental.

    **D. Criterion-based evaluation—YES, this is comparing performance to a criterion.**

27. An effective evaluation tool used to assess students' clinical understanding of patient care when they cannot be present is:

    **A. Case study—YES, case studies are often used as makeup clinical time.**

    B. Care plan—NO, this usually indicates there is patient interaction.

    C. Clinical skills checklist—NO, this needs to be demonstrated.

    D. Clinical evaluation rubric—NO, this is usually part of the actual clinical learning environment (CLE) assessment.

28. A nursing student makes a medication dosage error. The clinical nurse educator would:

    **A. Acknowledge the error.—YES, this is appropriate in a just culture.**

    B. Issue a clinical warning.—NO, this is not correct and reflects a blame versus just culture.

    C. Issue a failing grade.—NO, this is not correct and reflects a blame versus just culture.

    D. Report the student.—NO, this is not correct and reflects a blame culture versus just culture.

29. A clinical nurse educator faculty group is developing an evaluative instrument based on the course student learning outcomes (SLOs). This type of scale is most likely a:

    A. Case study—NO, this is usually complex patient information to simulate a real patient scenario.

    B. Care plan—NO, this usually calls for patient interaction.

    C. Clinical skills checklist—NO, this is procedural evaluation.

    **D. Clinical evaluation rubric—YES, this usually contains either standards or SLOs.**

30. One method used to decrease the subjectivity of a clinical evaluation instrument is to:

    A. Add criteria.—NO, although this makes the standards, or student learning outcomes (SLOs), more specific.

    B. Measure specific competencies.—NO, not just some need to be measured.

    C. Qualify the measures.—NO, this is too subjective.

    **D. Quantify the measures.—YES, this decreases subjectivity.**

31. The goal of a clinical evaluation is to ensure:

    A. The student has passed the courses—NO, this is part of a process of developing professional nurses.

    B. Ascertain what procedures have been completed—NO, this is evaluation criteria

    **C. Patient safety—YES, this is the ultimate goal.**

    D. Promote NCLEX success—NO, this is part of a process of developing professional nurses.

32. A clinical nurse educator would consider a student's repeated failure to turn in clinical assignments as:

    A. Lapsed behavior—NO, this is reckless behavior.

    B. At-risk behavior—NO, this is reckless behavior.

    **C. Reckless behavior—YES, this is correct.**

    D. Knowledge-based behavior—NO, this is reckless behavior.

33. Several nursing students approach the clinical nurse educator and inform her that a student is actively seeking and using opioids. The clinical nurse educator would take the following action:

    A. Allow the student to remain in the clinical area.—NO, patient safety is at stake as the student may have substance use or abuse.

    B. Change the student's clinical experience to an observation experience.—NO, the student's well-being is at stake as the student may have substance use or abuse.

C. Report the student to the nurse manager.—NO, the student's substance use or abuse would be addressed by the school.

**D. Confront the student about substance use.—YES, this is correct as the first step in managing substance use or abuse.**

34. The clinical nurse educator has a question regarding postclinical conference. She would consult which of the following?

    **A. Course faculty/coordinator—YES, the course faculty/coordinator would oversee and address this issue.**

    B. Department chair—NO, this is not the proper chain of command as the course/faculty or student would oversee and address this issue.

    C. Dean—NO, this is not the proper chain of command as the course/faculty or student would oversee and address this issue.

    D. Nurse manager—NO, this is not the proper chain of command as the course/faculty or student would oversee and address this issue.

35. A nursing student nearing program completion reaches out to a professor whom she felt was well respected in the professional nursing community. The student asks the professor to serve as a preceptor to her as she enters the workforce. The professor explains to the student that she would help her more as mentor versus a preceptor because:

    **A. A mentor relationship is one that does not have to carry over into the working environment but can last for several years.—YES, this is a valuable relationship that has already begun and can continue as peers, colleagues, and as a professional resource.**

    B. It is a professional obligation for all new nurses to have mentors from nursing school in order to socialize appropriately into the workforce.— NO, this is not a professional standard or requirement.

    C. A preceptor and a mentor are the same thing; however, professors can only serve as mentors.—No, preceptors and mentors have some commonalities; however, mentorship extends beyond a specific work environment.

    D. A preceptor and employee must sign a clinical contract for learning expectations and she cannot do this as nonemployee at another facility or institution.—No, this is not a mandatory professional guideline.

36. A nurse has recently completed her masters of science degree in nursing with a focus on education. She has worked as a bedside nurse on a medical-surgical nursing unit for the 3 years she has been a nurse and has been approached by her manager about being a unit-based educator for her peers, many of whom have been nurses for a much longer time than she has. In her new role, she finds that she is meeting resistance from her peers, who believe she is too young to be in the position. Her manager encourages her by reiterating the following statement regarding the nurse's clinical expertise:

    A. Her degree makes her the best person for the role.—NO, education does not equal solely clinical expertise.

    **B. Clinical expertise is a combination of accumulated knowledge through experience, formal education, and use of evidence that guides clinical**

decision-making.—YES, clinical expertise is developed over time but also consists of use of evidence and education.

   C. Even if she does not have the years of nursing experience, this position will help her develop her clinical expertise.—NO, this is not the best method to develop clinical skills.

   D. Nurses are known for "eating their young"; this is something she will just have to become accustomed to.—NO, an unjust culture should never be tolerated.

37. The nurse educator acknowledges that certification is important to her skill set because of which of the following?

   A. Certification increases salary.—NO, this may occur but is not always true.

   B. Certification is a requirement for clinical nurse educators.—NO, this may be an organizational goal but not a standardized requirement.

   **C. Certification is a method that clinical nurse educators use to validate their knowledge, skills, and experience beyond licensure.—YES, this is the intention of certification.**

   D. The clinical nurse educator certification is one that is intended for nurses working solely in academic settings.—NO, though this certification is often acquired by academic practitioners, the skills and knowledge that are validated are useful to a nurse in a practice setting as well.

38. The academic nursing program in which a nurse educator teaches does not focus on a single nursing theorist, but rather centers the curriculum around a combination of nursing theories. The educator learned *Orem's self-care deficit theory* as a nursing student and continues to exercise practice based on what she believes is derived from this theory. Which of the following concepts does she impress upon her students when caring for clients based on Orem's self-care deficit theory of nursing?

   **A. Encourage the client to actively participate in all activities of daily living (ADL) that they can.—YES, encourage clients to do what they can particularly while they are in your care and you can oversee their progress.**

   B. Teach the family to do all care-related tasks for the client.—NO, this does not foster self-care.

   C. Ensure nursing staff and assisting personnel are aware of client limitations and do not allow the patient to participate in care beyond this.—NO, understand limitations but encourage the client to work toward realistic goals.

   D. Avoid use of interdisciplinary services such as occupational or physical therapy.—NO, use as appropriate to help the client meet her or his goals.

39. The nurse educator encourages her students to participate in leadership opportunities that will most likely help them enhance their future leadership potential. Which of the following activities would be least likely to serve as a springboard for opportunities in leadership in nursing?

   A. Act as the team leader during clinical days.—NO, this provides opportunities to develop leadership characteristics.

B. Run for office in your academic program's student nurse association.—NO, this provides opportunities to develop leadership characteristics.

C. Join a nurses association in the state you plan to practice.—NO, this provides opportunities to develop leadership characteristics.

D. **Participate in a journal club.—YES, this primarily strengthens your research critique ability.**

40. A learner is struggling with care-plan sequencing in the clinical learning environment. The student tells the clinical nurse educator that he is an auditory learner. The clinical nurse educator can best assist him to understand the nursing process by:

A. Using a YouTube video.—NO, a YouTube video would be more effective for the person who is more of a visual learner or a mixed visual/auditory learner.

B. Switching to a concept map.—NO, a concept map is more effective for visual learners.

C. Have the student role-play what a nurse would do.—NO, role-playing is most effective for kinesthetic learners.

D. **Ask the student Socratic questions.—YES, Socratic questioning draws information from the student and allows him or her to think out loud.**

41. The nurse educator prepares an assignment for her clinical group. She asks the group to prioritize their patient list for rendering care. She instructs them to plan to assess the most critical patient first. What is the nurse educator trying to develop in the nursing student?

A. Personal growth—NO, that is not the main objective for the assignment.

B. Cultural awareness—NO, the type of patients are not described.

C. **Clinical decision-making—YES, this will help the student nurse in deciding which patient needs attention first.**

D. Exploration and understanding of their own beliefs and values—NO, this would be self-reflection.

42. A client admitted to a medical–surgical nursing floor has an implanted port that has been used to administer medications and obtain blood samples. The nurse educator demonstrates the process of obtaining a blood sample from the port to her students. The following week, the educator is notified that this patient has a double central line–associated bloodstream infection (CLABSI) and the hospital is performing a root cause analysis to determine a corrective action plan. The educator decides to share this scenario in a blind review as a case study with her students. She asks them to develop a mock action plan. What nursing skill is she trying to develop with these students?

A. **Clinical reasoning—YES, she has discovered an opportunity for her students to think through the process of how an adverse event occurred with this client.**

B. Correct process to draw blood—NO, this is understanding procedure.

C. Learning to avoid being part of a legal proceeding—NO, this is practicing within the scope of practice for a student.

D. Learning when to avoid using implanted ports—NO, this is not the objective of the learning experience.

43. The nurse educator prepares an assignment for her clinical group. She asks them to begin by developing a PICOT (patient/problem, intervention, comparison, outcome, time frame) question. She instructs them to learn the culture of the clinical unit and understand the patient population. Her desire is that they will, as a group, develop which of the following in order to give their project the momentum to achieve the best outcomes?

A. Personal relationships with the staff—NO, this is not the learning objective.

B. Cultural awareness—NO, this is not the learning objective.

C. **A spirit of inquiry—YES, this is necessary in order to move the evidence-based practice (EBP) process forward; all the other options are helpful but this group needs to have a spirit of inquiry to cultivate the best outcomes.**

D. Exploration and understanding of their own beliefs and values—NO, this is not the learning objective.

44. The role of the clinical nurse specialist has changed and/or been eliminated over time largely due to a business model that ultimately eliminated the economic value of the role. Nursing has a large responsibility to advocate for this role because it supports client-driven outcomes that create positive health outcomes. This involves integrating best practices with which of the following?

A. **Clinical expertise and patient preference—YES, these help the nurse provides the client more comprehensive care.**

B. Personal experience and the clients' socioeconomic status—NO, socioeconomics of the patient should not be the consideration.

C. Research utilization and policy review—NO, this is not the objective.

D. The nurses' experience and education level—NO, this is not the most salient factor.

45. Evidence demonstrates that student satisfaction is increased when clinical nurse educators are:

A. Personable to students—NO, this is not the major attribute that contributes to student satisfaction.

B. Good delegators—NO, this is not the major attribute that contributes to student satisfaction.

C. **Organized—YES, students appreciate organization and feel that it increases the effectiveness of the learning environment.**

D. Friendly with staff—NO, this is not the major attribute that contributes to student satisfaction.

46. The clinical nurse educator has a responsibility to balance student and patient needs. She can best do this by incorporating a model or set of competencies that create a framework for meeting these objectives. Which competency will help the educator balance her responsibilities?

A. Value-based care—NO, this is not a Quality and Safety Education for Nurses (QSEN) competency.

B. Family-centered care—No, this does not address patient needs.

C. **Quality improvement—YES, this is a QSEN competency.**

D. Clinical preference—NO, this does not address patient needs.

47. The clinical nurse educator is assisting students in performing health assessments and health histories. The primary objective for today's assignment is to develop the students' ability to obtain a more thorough and detailed focused assessment. The optimal method to teach then would be:

A. **Asking open-ended questions—YES, by asking open-ended type of questions, the student can obtain more information and allows for further elaboration.**

B. Asking yes or no questions—NO, the more appropriate questions are open ended.

C. Performing tests—NO, it may be appropriate to obtain test results; however, when conversing with the patient, it is important for students to ask open-ended questions.

D. Seeing what the healthcare provider has documented—NO, even though one may want to compare findings, it is important for students to learn how to obtain histories and develop techniques.

48. Discussing with students different viewpoints, perspectives, and ideas across disciplines is an ideal way to build:

A. Cultural competence—NO, cultural competence is built on understanding different ways of life.

B. **Collaboration—YES, when applied across disciplines this creates collaboration.**

C. Diversity—NO, it really builds an understanding of collaboration.

D. Communication—NO, communication is an aspect of creating collaboration across disciplines.

49. Nursing students should be taught that evidence-based research has determined that using this skill reduces preventable healthcare errors:

A. Critical thinking—NO, even though this skill is crucial, the majority of preventable healthcare errors is caused by lack of communication.

B. Collaboration—NO, communication is the key component of collaboration.

C. Self-reflection—NO, self-reflection is a key component in analyzing one's communication skills.

D. **Communication—YES, when this skill is practiced and implemented with tools, evidence has demonstrated a reduction in preventable healthcare errors.**

50. It is imperative to reduce and eliminate incivility in the workplace, as it can create issues that impact both the staff and the patient. As the clinical nurse educator, you realize the main component to emphasize when educating students is:

A. Communication—NO, this is an essential component, but the best manner to resolve this is to initiate conflict management, so students can realize the impact this creates.

B. Collaborative practice—NO, once conflict management is done, collaboration should result.

C. **Conflict management—YES, this is needed to assist students to realize the impact incivility has on the work environment.**

D. Self-reflection—NO, despite the students needing to practice self-reflection to realize the negative impact incivility has, the crucial component to implement is conflict management.

51. The clinical nurse educator is explaining to the clinical group that when one's values and ethics are not congruent with the organizations' values and ethics, a resulting effect may be:

A. **Internal conflict—YES, internal conflict is created when personal ethics and values are compromised.**

B. Organizational conflict—NO, it is possible to have organizational conflict if there is misalignment of ethics and values, but it will usually result in personal internal conflict.

C. Personal alignment of their ethics to those of the organization—NO, one should remain true to oneself, as stated in the *Code of Ethics* and which is called *maintaining authenticity*.

D. It does not create any conflict—NO, when there is no alignment, conflict is created.

52. An intrinsic factor that motivates clinical nurse educators to certification is:

A. Merit awards from employers—NO, this is an extrinsic motivator.

B. Rank promotion—NO, this is an extrinsic motivator.

C. **Building confidence—YES, this is intrinsic and something one does for themselves.**

D. Recognition by national organizations—NO, this is an extrinsic motivator.

53. While making rounds on the clinical nurse educator's assigned area, the clinical nurse educator brings a particular staff member to the clinical director's attention because this person has been engaging in inappropriate conversation with several healthcare providers. As the clinical nurse educator, you should:

A. Actively listen to environmental surroundings.—NO, this is one of the first important steps in conflict management, by being vigilant in assessing the environment. However, you have proceeded to the next step.

B. Remain calm.—NO, this is an important component of conflict management, but not in this situation.

C. Recognize conflict early.—NO, this is one of the first important steps in conflict management, by being vigilant in assessing the environment. However, you have proceeded to the next step.

D. **Be proactive.—YES, this is the second step of conflict management; and taking this to the Clinical Director is being proactive.**

54. While conducting conflict management skill-building scenarios with your students, it is important to emphasize:

   A. Utilize "you" statements.—NO, utilizing this type of statement may put the other person on the defensive.

   B. **Utilize "I" statements.—YES, utilizing this type of statement brings the feelings surrounding the issue back on the person initiating the conversation, instead of placing blame and putting the other person on the defensive.**

   C. Place blame.—NO, placing blame does not resolve the conflict, and puts others on the defensive.

   D. Avoid the situation.—NO, avoiding the situation will only make the situation worse and not resolve matters.

55. It is essential for future professional nurses to develop this skill in order to effectively manage patient care through collaborative practice:

   A. **Leadership—YES, this is an important skill set to use to work collaboratively with other disciplines. This is reinforced by the Institute of Medicine.**

   B. Evidence-based practice—NO, evidence has shown that leadership skills build collaborative skills.

   C. Delegation—NO, this skill does not build collaboration with other disciplines.

   D. Prioritization—NO, this skill does not build collaboration with other disciplines.

56. Practicing collaboration builds on an important component(s), which is (are):

   A. Critical thinking—NO, critical thinking is used in collaborative practice, but is not necessarily needed as a main aspect of collaborative practice.

   B. Experience—NO, experience will aid in developing collaborative practice but is not the main aspect.

   C. Quality and safety—NO, this is an outcome of collaborative practice.

   D. **Trust and respect—YES, this is a crucial component of effective collaborative teams.**

57. While conducting strategies to resolve a conflict, a student member begins directing volatile comments at you. The best strategy for the clinical nurse educator to utilize is:

   A. Get up and leave.—NO, the best strategy to utilize is to attempt to keep one's emotions in check and remain calm.

   B. Return the volatile comments.—NO, this will not solve anything, but it will make matters worse.

   C. **Remain calm.—YES, this is the best tactic to employ. The student is possibly attempting to divert attention from himself or herself. Remaining calm is a primary objective of conflict resolution.**

   D. Let someone else deal with this.—NO, it is important to deal with conflict appropriately as a role model.

**58.** A student is talking at lunch about his family putting pressure on him to attend family events when he needs to be studying. What response by the clinical nurse educator would be most helpful?

    A. "Students usually have to put their social life on hold while in the nursing program."—NO, students may need to reduce their attendance at social events, but should not eliminate them.

    B. "You will need to tell your family that school is your priority now."—NO, the family remains an important support system for the student.

    C. "Tell your family that you are not feeling well and are unable to attend."—NO, the clinical nurse educator should not advocate for dishonesty.

    **D. "Let's talk about some time-management skills that may be helpful to you."—YES, this is a solution that can assist the student in managing school and family more effectively.**

**59.** The clinical nurse educator notices that a student is quiet and isolated from the other students. After being asked whether anything was wrong, the student states that she feels that she has no connection to anyone and is questioning her career choice. What action by the clinical nurse educator would be most helpful?

    A. Send the student for counseling.—NO, this would be appropriate if the student seems depressed, but may not address the issue.

    B. Assign another student to work with her.—NO, this would be forcing a relationship that may not be helpful.

    **C. Identify a mentor willing to work with the student.—YES, a mentor can be supportive and provide guidance to the student as she adapts to the nursing profession.**

    D. Recommend that she speak to a university guidance counselor.—NO, it would be premature to assume the student wants to change her major.

**60.** A clinical nurse educator is using strategies to encourage clinical decision-making. What action by the educator would best facilitate this?

    **A. Ask questions throughout the clinical day.—YES, Socratic questioning and asking the question why encourages critical thinking.**

    B. Demonstrate skills before allowing students to perform them.—NO, observation is not as effective in promoting clinical decision-making.

    C. Provide explanations for complex patient care issues.—NO, this provides the student with the answers, but does not encourage individual thought.

    D. Encourage the students to observe the nurses in critical situations.—NO, observation is not as effective in promoting clinical decision-making.

**61.** A clinical group is composed of eight multigenerational students. Which teaching–learning strategy would be most effective with this group?

    A. Lecture on a complex diagnosis during postconference.—NO, this is teacher-directed and most effective for baby boomers.

    B. Assign a group project to be completed in postconference.—NO, although group projects can be beneficial, many students do not prefer this strategy.

C. **Utilize a variety of methods based on student response.—YES, a variety of strategies are effective for the greatest number of students.**

D. Require students to use smartphones to identify best practices.—NO, millennials are the most comfortable with technology.

62. One prominent reason there is an increased social need for clinical nurse educators is:

A. **There is an increased need for nurses due to baby boomers living longer.—YES, there are more healthcare needs in the United States.**

B. Nurses do not stay at the bedside.—NO, this is a factor but not a prominent reason.

C. There are more second-degree nursing students who are older.—NO, many students are still seeking first degrees.

D. Many clinical nurse educators team teach students.—NO, this is not the reason.

63. A student informs her clinical nurse educator that the nurse she is working with is not answering questions and acts as though the student is an annoyance. How should the clinical nurse educator first respond?

A. Remove the student from this nurse's assignment.—NO, this is premature before seeking further information.

B. Speak with the nurse manager about the nurse's behavior.—NO, the problem should first be addressed with the nurse involved.

C. **Discuss student responsibilities with the nurse and her expectations.— YES, it is important to open communication with the nurse and attempt to resolve the issue.**

D. Question the student's interpretation of the nurse's behavior.—NO, this conveys mistrust and will likely block the student from reporting future incidents.

64. An experienced clinical nurse educator is describing the importance of facilitating the learners' understanding of the consequences of their actions following a simulation scenario. This technique is an example of:

A. Active learning—NO, this is a method of teaching/learning in which learners are engaged in the instruction.

B. **Reflective debriefing—YES, this is a structured process that guides learners to connect the events of the situation to the outcomes.**

C. Constructive feedback—NO, this is providing feedback that is honest, yet tactful and helpful to the learner.

D. Problem solving—NO, this is an organized method for finding solutions to problems.

65. Students are found to be taking selfies with their smartphones in the nurses' station. Which response by the clinical nurse educator would be best in this situation?

A. "This could be grounds for you all being dismissed from the nursing program."—NO, this may be an accurate statement but scare tactics are not usually effective.

B. "You need to put away your phones before you are caught doing this."—NO, this carries the meaning that the educator is covering for the students.

C. "You have been told that you cannot take pictures while in clinical."—NO, this provides no information on what is being done wrong.

D. **"This could be a breach of patient confidentiality if a name is seen in a picture."—YES, this connects the students' action with a direct consequence that has the potential to harm the patient; this should have an impact on the students.**

66. A learner is struggling with care-plan sequencing in the clinical learning environment. The student tells the clinical nurse educator that he is a visual learner. The clinical nurse educator can best assist him to understand the nursing process by:

A. Using a YouTube video—NO, this is not the best learning tool for the nursing process.

B. **Switching to a concept map—YES, this can assist a visual learner to make the process links.**

C. Have him role-play what a nurse would do—NO, this would be better for a kinesthetic learner.

D. Ask him Socratic questions—NO, this would be better for a verbal learner.

67. The clinical nurse educator overhears staff nurses laughing and disparaging a patient within hearing of several students. What is the educator's best response?

A. Ignore the behavior as harmless.—NO, these are not the professional behaviors expected of nurses.

B. Inform the nurse manager of the incident.—NO, the incident should first be addressed with the people involved.

C. **Discuss the incident in postconference.—YES, students need to understand that this behavior is unprofessional and nurses are often looked to as role models.**

D. Confront the nurses about their behavior.—NO, this may need to be addressed at some point, but the educator's priority is the students.

68. A novice clinical nurse educator tells her mentor that she works very hard to be tolerant of the differences of diverse individuals. What would be the mentor's best response?

A. **"It is important to work toward embracing differences rather than tolerating them."—YES, in working toward a clinical learning environment of inclusive excellence, it is important to see differences as bringing added value.**

B. "Demonstrating tolerance is important in helping people to feel accepted."—NO, the goal of the clinical nurse educator is to encourage inclusive excellence, which goes beyond tolerance.

C. "There are some students who are very difficult to like."—NO, this is not appropriate.

D. "You need to be fair to everyone so that no one feels discriminated against."—NO, this is not a helpful statement.

69. Following a patient code on the unit, students witness the clinical nurse educator assisting the unlicensed assistive personnel (UAP) to provide postmortem care before the family arrives. This is an example of:

    A. Mentoring the UAP—NO, there is no evidence of mentoring occurring in this situation.

    B. Educating the UAP—NO, there is no evidence of education in this scenario.

    **C. Modeling teamwork—YES, this is an example of unconscious role-modeling of a positive professional behavior.**

    D. Empathizing with the UAP—NO, there is no evidence that the clinical nurse educator is demonstrating empathy.

70. When asking learners to choose an intervention related to a medication's side effect, the clinical nurse educator is using what level of Bloom's taxonomy?

    A. Understanding—NO, this is recall.

    **B. Application—YES, this is choosing an appropriate intervention.**

    C. Comprehension—NO, this is understanding why it happened.

    D. Creating—NO, this is coming up with something new.

71. Many nurses learned about nursing care through on-the-job training. The type of learner who learns best with hands-on experience through clinical practice uses what type of learning style?

    A. Visual learner—NO, these learners prefer visual clues such as graphics.

    B. Audio learner—NO, these learners prefer to hear instructions.

    **C. Kinesthetic learner—YES, these are hands-on learners.**

    D. Multimodal learner—NO, these learners can use more than one learning method and can switch as needed.

72. Nurse educators who use a pedagogical approach to facilitate learners in an active style of teaching expect the students to:

    **A. Become involved in doing and thinking about what they are doing.—YES, this is engagement in learning.**

    B. Participate in lecturing in the class.—NO, this is passive.

    C. Be diligent in taking notes in class.—NO, this is passive.

    D. Be ready to look up answers on their smartphones while listening in class.—NO, this is active, but is only one methodology and not the overall concept of active learning..

73. Clinical nurse educators know working in the clinical setting can be very stressful for students. One method the nurse educator can use to reduce that stress and enhance student learning is to do which of the following?

    A. Leave the unit and let the floor nurse monitor the student's activities.—NO, the clinical nurse educator's presence will reduce stress.

B. Use humor appropriately and mindfulness training prior to patient care.—YES, this can help reduce stress if used appropriately.

C. Allow the student to work more autonomously.—NO, students need guidance.

D. Allow the student to make small mistakes and correct them in postconference.—NO, anticipate the learner's needs.

74. The clinical nurse educator will be bringing a new group of students to a new clinical site. The clinical nurse educator realizes the students will have enhanced learning under which of the following conditions?

A. The nursing staff works closely with the faculty and is aware of the learning outcomes.—YES, this helps the learning environment.

B. The nursing staff were former graduates of the school of nursing and knows what to expect.—NO, this is not always the best way to prepare a culture of learning.

C. The nurse educator is completely in control of all nursing student activities.—NO, collaborating and communicating create a rich learning environment.

D. Nursing staff only assign to students those patients who pose no real challenge to cause any disruptions in healthcare.—NO, this does not allow students to learn new skills.

75. Clinical nurse educators who teach in the clinical setting realize evidence-based research is essential to teaching students how to:

A. Focus on critical thinking and clinical reasoning.—YES, this helps students make good clinical decisions.

B. Never deviate from hospital-approved clinical pathways.—NO, this is done sometimes to personalize care.

C. Always consult the clinical protocols before performing a procedure.—NO, sometimes there is not time and a decision must be made.

D. Consider using the tried-and-true methods of healthcare treatments.—NO, tradition does not always dictate the most efficient and effective care.

76. Clinical nurse educators know critical thinking skills enhance the students' abilities to do which of the following?

A. Process information, problem-solve, and make judgments.—YES, this enhances the quality of nursing care.

B. Know what to do in any given situation all the time.—NO, this is impossible for one nurse or person to know.

C. Create a care plan that can be used universally for most patients.—NO, care plans need personalization to be effective.

D. Follow the same routine daily without deviation.—NO, care needs personalization and continuous reevaluation to be effective.

77. A clinical setting is conducive to learning when the student is able to do which of the following?

A. Work independently without interference from the staff.—NO, staff are role models and mentors also.

B. **Work with the staff who accepts the student with a positive attitude.— YES, this produces the best learning environments.**

C. Have an opportunity to meet the staff at an informal greeting outside of the clinic.—NO, this is nice, but not necessary.

D. Have relatives who work in the healthcare profession at another clinic.— NO, this is not necessary.

78. The clinical nurse educator is teaching a group of students about cultural competence. The students understand what cultural competence is when:

A. The student mimics someone else's culture and practices to make that person feel at home.—NO, the learner does not have to pretend to display the patient's cultural habits.

B. The student asks the patient to explain why the patient believes in that culture.—NO, this is confrontational.

C. **The student understands the unique needs and preferences of ethnic minorities without changing his or her own beliefs.—YES, this is respect for the patient and self.**

D. The student expects others to change to follow current local customs now they are no longer in their country.—NO, this is disrespectful and unrealistic.

79. Clinical nurse educators are always interested in bringing in new technology and strategies to teach students. Which of the following would be considered an active method of teaching to enhance clinical competencies?

A. Have a guest speaker who is an expert in his or her field present to the class.—NO, this may not include technology.

B. Have the students participate in a field trip to a specialized clinic to observe new experiences.—NO, this is passive learning.

C. **Incorporate simulation-based clinical experiences for the student in a controlled and safe environment.—YES, this will assist learning.**

D. Have the students present previously learned clinical experiences in class.—NO, this does not encourage new knowledge.

80. Which of the following is the best assignment to help learners use evidence-based practice to improve clinical safety?

A. **Ask learners to identify a safety issue in clinical practice and have them research evidence-based practices related to this issue.—YES, by actively engaging in a real-time practice experience assignment, learners will acquire more knowledge.**

B. Ask learners to read an article about clinical safety and evidence-based practices.—NO, this is passive learning, which can hinder the amount of knowledge one will obtain.

C. Show the learners a video about clinical safety and evidence-based practices.—NO, simply watching a video is not actively engaging the learners.

    D. Lead a class discussion about clinical safety and evidence-based practices.—NO, although this is actively engaging students, not all students may participate and/or it is not being correlated into a practical clinical situation.

81. Which of the following is considered an intrinsic motivator that could be the reason why a candidate is seeking certification?

    A. Maintaining employment—NO, this is an extrinsic motivator. May need certification to keep your current position.

    B. Career advancement—NO, this is an extrinsic motivator. May help get a job promotion.

    C. Financial incentive—No, this is an extrinsic motivator. May be able to negotiate a better salary.

    **D. Sense of accomplishment—YES, this is an intrinsic motivator. Comes from desire to achieve, values, and personal satisfaction.**

82. The nurse educator has asked learners to do a concept map of a patient's care plan but finds that some learners are having difficulty creating this map. Which type of learner is most likely to construct a well-created map?

    **A. Visual—YES, they learn best by using diagrams, illustrations, symbols, and maps.**

    B. Kinesthetic—NO, they learn best by a hands-on approach or watching a live demonstration.

    C. Auditory—NO, they learn best by reading aloud, group discussion, or quizzing fellow students.

    D. Read/Write—NO, they learn best through words, such as rewriting material over in their own way to enhance their understanding.

83. Working with learners in the clinical setting provides the benefit of evaluating which type of learning that is difficult to evaluate in the classroom setting?

    A. Cognitive—NO, this can be evaluated both within the clinical and classroom settings.

    **B. Psychomotor—YES, this is demonstration of skills and the clinical nurse educator can easily observe these being carried out during patient care.**

    C. Affective—NO, this can be evaluated within the clinical and classroom settings.

    D. Moral—NO, this is a subcategory of the affective domain.

84. Which is an accurate statement related to studying within a group?

    A. No leader should be identified in order to be sure all group members are considered equal.—NO, someone should be appointed to lead the discussion and to be sure everyone stays focused and does not get off-task.

    B. There should be a start time but the study session should continue until all learners feel it is time to stop.—NO, there should be both a determined start and stop time to maintain structure.

C. Breaks should be taken whenever the learners feel overwhelmed or fatigued.—NO, breaks are important to include but they should be planned when and how long they should last.

D. **A set topic to discuss that day should be established with clear outcomes.—YES, this is vital so that everyone is committed to reaching the same outcomes. Guidelines are important to formulate so the discussion stays on track.**

85. What cognitive level, from Bloom's Taxonomy, does the following question fit: "You have just received your patient's electrolyte results and note the potassium is 3.2 mEq/L. What nursing interventions are needed?"

A. Knowledge—NO, this question is asking what should be done about a particular problem. It is more complex than a knowledge (recall) question.

B. Comprehension—NO, the question is asking one to apply what knowledge they possess to a particular situation. The question is more complex than comprehending information.

C. **Application—YES, this question is expecting the learner to provide an intervention to a problem based on applying concepts and principles to a situation.**

D. Evaluation—NO, the intervention has not been implemented; therefore, it would be difficult to determine if it was effective or ineffective.

86. When one experiences test anxiety, a coping strategy to employ would be to have the person

A. Arrive at the testing center 5 minutes before the test begins to avoid hearing others talk about the exam.—NO, it is important to arrive 15 minutes early so that you do not feel rushed. Do a trial drive to the exam center to help identify the time it takes to arrive.

B. Perform a last-minute review the evening prior to the scheduled exam.—NO, this will only increase anxiety as one begins to doubt themselves and feel they are not ready.

C. **Carry out deep breathing techniques and guided imagery.—YES, concentrating on relaxation techniques can help clear one's mind as well as promote a calmness.**

D. Tell yourself that you have never been a great test-taker and not to expect the best.—NO, negative self-talk can disrupt your focus and performance. Replace negative thoughts with positive ones that can serve as motivators.

87. It is the evening before the candidate's scheduled exam. What would be the most beneficial way to spend this evening?

A. Go out to a nightclub for drinks and dancing with friends.—NO, drinking alcohol can cause one to inadvertently sleep later than desired or can interrupt sleep. Engaging in aerobic activities, such as dancing, prior to going to bed, could affect one's ability to fall asleep.

B. Stay up as late as possible to continue studying the weak content areas.—NO, adequate sleep is positively correlated to academic performance. Lack of sleep can contribute to the inability to recall specific topics and can interfere with one's level of concentration.

C. Spend the evening at home with family watching movies.—YES, it is crucial that one spend time with family and/or friends (socialization is important for emotional health). Engaging in enjoyable activities will promote relaxation.

D. Spend time on the phone talking to a friend who is complaining about her boyfriend—NO, this scenario could put you in a negative mood and increase tension levels.

88. The clinical nurse educator is role-modeling the importance of interprofessional communication and collaboration while on the clinical unit. Which National League for Nursing (NLN) core competency is this nurse educator exhibiting?

A. Functioning as a change agent and leader—YES, promoting and valuing interprofessional collaboration allows the learners to see that a shared learning environment exists. In addition, this collaboration helps to address certain healthcare and educational needs.

B. Pursuing continuous quality improvement in the nurse educator role— NO, this competency ensures that learners are provided opportunities for professional development.

C. Engaging in scholarship—NO, clinical nurse educators must make a commitment to lifelong learning and to remain aware of the most current evidence-based practice guidelines.

D. Facilitating learner development and socialization—NO, opportunities to emphasize professionalism, integrity, respect, and accountability of the learners fall into this competency. Incorporating cultural beliefs is also a crucial component.

89. Which of the following statements is true related to the Certified Academic Clinical Nurse Educator (CNE®cl) certification examination?

A. Every question on the examination counts toward your overall score.— NO, there are 20 question items that do not count toward the candidate's score. These are questions that are incorporated into the exam to obtain statistics to see whether or not they can be used in future exams. The candidate does not know which ones are pretest or operational.

B. It is composed mainly of low-level thinking items since they emphasize specific details.—NO, these exams are mainly composed of high-level thinking items. They require a deeper understanding of principles and concepts.

C. Items are written by a select few nurse educators from one type of program located within a small geographical range.—NO, exam items are developed by numerous academic nurse educators from a variety of program types spanning a large geographical area.

D. It relies heavily on forming associations among various concepts and applying knowledge in a contextual manner.—YES, certification exams are more global in nature when compared to course exams. They do not rely on simply recalling facts/details.

**90.** The best method for the clinical nurse educator to validate her or his skills is to

A. Develop policies and procedures.—NO, although this demonstrates expertise it may not validate all skills.

B. Contribute to didactic test questions.—NO, although this demonstrates expertise it is usually specific to the course faculty.

C. Work as staff on the unit they teach.—NO, working does not necessarily validate all skills.

**D. Obtain certification.—YES, this is a great method to validate skill.**

**91.** A student states that he believes that the patient's cancer was caused by environmental chemicals. The clinical nurse educator asks the student to describe the type of cancer and then to make the link from the environmental chemical to the pathology. This type of coaching can be considered

A. Direct questioning—NO, this elicits a yes or no answer.

B. Reflection—NO, this is not about the student's feelings.

**C. Scaffolding—YES, this encourages students to think of the next step.**

D. Care planning—NO, this is a process for nursing care.

**92.** The clinical nurse educator has a good understanding of student preparedness when he states

**A. "I will ask them to discuss their patients in preconference."—YES, this is a good method to assess preparedness.**

B. "I will administer a quiz before they start the day."—NO, this is not a method that can encompass all patient types that the students will care for.

C. "The staff nurse will tell them what they need to know for their patients."—NO, this is not the staff's responsibility.

D. "Only the patient's main diagnosis should be addressed in the care plan initially."—NO, this is not holistic patient education.

**93.** A novice clinical nurse educator when dealing with a student who fails clinically needs additional understanding of "due process" when she states

A. "I have provided the student with a warning about her poor performance before the failure."—NO, this is the correct thing to do to warn the student.

**B. "The student should understand that she has been consistently performing poorly."—YES, there needs to be documentation that the student has been told.**

C. "The student did not follow the plan for improvement as signed."—NO, this is the correct thing to do to warn the student.

D. "The student was told on multiple occasions that without improvement this would be a course failure."—NO, this is the correct thing to do to warn the student.

**94.** The novice clinical nurse educator needs additional understanding of evidence-based clinical teaching practice when he states

A. "The acute care center that is Magnet recognized may offer more learning opportunities."—NO, this may be true because nursing may have more autonomy.

**B. "I have made sure that all students are at the same place each semester for continuity."—YES, multiple opportunities demonstrate better learning outcomes.**

C. "The 'nursing home' is not a good place for students to learn skills."—NO, this may be a very good place to learn holistic care and skills are done at many long-term care facilities.

D. "Assessing the clinical environment culture is important for learning opportunities."—NO, this is definitely needed to ensure learning.

95. One method of ensuring that students have the most up-to-date evidence to base their patient care decisions in the clinical learning environment (CLE) is to use

A. Textbooks that are less than 5 years old—NO, evidence changes faster than a 5-year time span.

B. Journal articles less than 5 years old—NO, evidence changes faster than a 5-year time span.

C. The healthcare organization's policies—NO, these are only updated at intervals.

**D. A mobile app designed for reference—YES, these are consistently updated.**

96. One of the reasons for high attrition rates for graduate nurses is

A. Lack of physical skill attainment—NO, this is usually not the cause.

B. Decreasing pay scales—NO, this is not the main cause.

C. Overmentoring—NO, this increases retention.

**D. Lack of judgment ability—YES, this has been noted by nurse administrators.**

97. A method to assist the novice clinical nurse educator fulfill the role is to

A. Have the educator take an academic nursing education course.—NO, this may not be clinical education based.

**B. Provide the educator a mentor to observe.—YES, this is a good way to orientate them to the role.**

C. Tell the educator to use his or her clinical experience as a guide.—NO, experience as a practicing RN does not provide the knowledge necessary for the role of clinical nursing educator.

D. Instruct the educator to match the students with staff nurses.—NO, the clinical nurse educator is ultimately responsible for facilitating the teaching/learning of the nursing students.

98. An undergraduate nursing student passes out in the clinical area and is not hurt. The stat tells the clinical nurse educator that she did not eat. The clinical nurse educator should first

A. Provide her with a snack—NO, this can be done but she should be checked first.

B. Call her parents to come get her.—NO, this may be a Health Insurance Portability and Accountability Act (HIPAA) violation.

**C. Have her taken to the emergency room.—YES, she should be checked.**

D. Notify the course coordinator.—NO, this can be done second.

99. The novice clinical nurse educator needs better understanding of the concept of integrity when he states, "Integrity includes:

A. Honesty."—NO, this is an attribute of integrity.

B. Ethical behavior."—NO, this is an attribute of integrity.

**C. Role modeling"—YES, this is not an attribute and although the clinical nurse educator should role-model integrity it is not a given.**

D. Professionalism"—NO, this is an attribute of integrity.

100. An effective method to teach students leadership in the clinical learning environment (CLE) is

A. Have them shadow the nurse manager.—NO, this is not the most effective method.

B. Have them make assignments.—NO, this is a managerial task.

C. Ask them to teach a group of patients.—NO, teaching is every nurse's role.

**D. Have them role-model being in charge.—YES, this will assist them to understand how to be a leader.**

# Index

Printed in the United States
By Bookmasters